Wanting Another Child

Coping with Secondary Infertility

Harriet Fishman Simons

LEXINGTON BOOKS
An Imprint of The Free Press
NEW YORK   LONDON   TORONTO   SYDNEY   TOKYO   SINGAPORE

Library of Congress Cataloging-in-Publication Data

Simons, Harriet Fishman
    Wanting another child : coping with secondary infertility /
Harriet Fishman Simons.
        p.   cm.
    Includes bibliographical references.
    ISBN 0–02–928938–6
    1. Infertility.   2. Infertility—Psychological aspects.
I. Title
RC889.S56   1995
616.6'92—dc20   94–41404
                                                         CIP

Lexington Books
An Imprint of The Free Press
A Division of Simon & Schuster Inc.
866 Third Avenue, New York, N. Y. 10022

Printed in the United States of America

printing number

1 2 3 4 5 6 7 8 9 10

For My Family

I wish I had as many children as Mrs. Walesa.

—Hillary Rodham Clinton
quoted by the Associated Press,
July 8, 1994

Contents

Acknowledgments

The publication of this book marks twenty years of my involvement with infertility: at first, personally, as I experienced recurring infertility and pregnancy loss and, later, professionally, as I became an infertility therapist, researcher/writer, and RESOLVE support group leader.

One of the positive outcomes of infertility for me is the people I have met during these years. I owe a great deal to those who helped me during my own journey through infertility. I will always be grateful to the member of a women's support group in which I participated in 1978—to Barbara Eck Menning, founder of RESOLVE, and Peg Cramer, RESOLVE's first Chair. I was privileged to serve on the National RESOLVE Board from 1979 to 1989 and also on the Board of RESOLVE of the Bay State, which enabled me to get to know others who cared deeply about infertility.

I have also had the opportunity to work with and learn from other support group leaders and members of the National and Bay State Clinical Advisory Committees, professionals dedicated to helping those experiencing infertility. The ongoing exchange of insights and perspectives with my colleagues and the relationships I have formed with them have enriched me both professionally and personally. I would like to specifically thank Peg Beck, Executive Director of RESOLVE of the Bay State, and Merle Bombardieri, RESOLVE of the Bay State support group supervisor, for their help over the years.

I am most grateful to my clients and group members who have shared their experiences with me and in this way have informed my thinking and deepened my understanding of secondary infertility. While their stories have not been cited in this book nor have they been acknowledged by name, their desire that others understand the pain of secondary infertility motivated me to write this book.

I would like to thank the editors of RESOLVE and Stepping Stones Newsletters for graciously printing my request for first-hand accounts of secondary infertility. I would also like to thank Diane Aronson, Executive Director of National RESOLVE; Ron Porter Good, Executive Director, Parents of Only Children; Janet Lawn, Field Director, National RESOLVE; and Patricia McShane, M.D. Medical Director of IVF–America for their assistance.

The individuals who shared their stories with me gave this book its heart. I am deeply impressed and touched by their generosity and desire that others escape the isolation so many of them have experienced. While it is impossible to do justice to the richness and complexity of each individual's situation, I hope that this book reflects their collective experience. I would like to thank the following people as well as those who prefer not to be acknowledged by name for their openness, insight, and interest in this project: Sue Alfiero, Cheryl Amspan, Pamela Balus, Margaret Barsalou, Melanie Birchfield, B. Lynn and Nadine Boehm, Peggy Burke, Karen Christenson, Lois Clas, Susan Cohen, Joan Collins, Julie Cornett, Gina Cousineau, Lisa Couver, Glenda Croak, Valerie Dehrhe, Donna Demarest, Maribeth Dunlavy, Kimberly Edwards, Lisa Kehayias-Farhi, Carolyn Fine, Jane Fisher, Susan Florez, Janet Gilligan, Deborah Goodman, Teddi Lyn Guffy, Carol Ann Hill, Nancy Holloway, Jean Hoffman, Lori and Jeff Kenney, Denise Landmesser, Pam Levine, Jodie Linger, Barbara Luker, Noreen McGowan, Renee Larry, Beth McKeown, Jacqueline Mitchell, Linda Neuenhaus, Sally Odhner, Susan Page, Bonnie Penner, Denise Platt, Fern Rabinovitz, Sandy Raia, Roxie Shaul, Ellen Speyer, Deb Steeler, Lisa Travis, Valerie Van Hollen, Jana Whatley, Dana Zinderman, Ruth Zschoche, Judith Zvara.

I am most appreciative of the significant contributions to this book made by those who read earlier drafts of specific chapters and/or the entire manuscript. Their comments made this book better than it would otherwise have been. (Any remaining shortcomings are solely my own.) This group helped me in numerous ways by generously providing encouragement, frank criticism, advice, painstaking critiques, and a wealth of personal insight and clinical expertise. A most heartfelt thank you to Karen Berkeley, Judith

Calica, Diane Clapp, James Drisko, Geri Ferber, Patricia Johnston, Miriam Mazor, M.D., and Liz Raab.

This book would not have been undertaken without the encouragement, prodding, and example of my colleague Aline Zoldbrod who preceded me down the road to publishing, and without my husband Steven's confidence that I could (and should) write a book. I would like to thank my children, Sara, Rebecca, and David, who gave up computer time, helped me find my eyeglasses, sharpened pencils, and cheerfully ate pizzas and Chinese take-out food for dinner. Their very existence provides a personal context for this book. I would also like to thank my relatives and friends for their ongoing assistance and caring.

Finally, I would like to thank my editor, Margaret Zusky, who not only provided editorial feedback but also managed to find me a much needed babysitter when school was out and my deadline was fast approaching!

Wanting Another Child

1

An Overview of
Secondary Infertility

I didn't think that infertility applied to me.

—Woman who had tried for years to give birth to another child

The past fifteen to twenty years have brought a growing awareness of the pain of infertility that previously existed as an invisible loss. Yet despite the attention recently paid to infertility in general, infertility following the birth of a child (or children) remains the hidden form of infertility. Secondary infertility seems to be in the same place where infertility was two decades ago: still "in the closet" and unaddressed.

Infertility can and does follow successful pregnancies; past fertility is no guarantee for the future. Even if you once conceived easily or even without trying, you may have found yourself, perhaps after a few years of conscientiously attempting to space your children, despairing as to whether you will be able to have more children at all. If you hoped that the birth of your child signaled the end of infertility in your life, you may subsequently have learned that rather than having been "cured," you must once again confront this problem.

Infertility among parents feels different from infertility among the childless. Each situation is painful and has unique dynamics. The intent here is not to compare or rank the losses, but rather to explore and validate what is a very real loss: the loss of the full family for which you have longed.

Defining Secondary Infertility

Many couples who are suffering from secondary infertility do not know there even is such a condition, let alone what they can do about it. Medically, the phrase "secondary infertility" has generally been used to refer to couples who are unable to conceive but previously were able to establish pregnancies, whereas "primary infertility" refers to couples who have never been able to achieve a pregnancy.[1]

For the purposes of this book, however, I prefer a definition that is both broader and narrower. In my view, secondary infertility is the inability to conceive a pregnancy *or carry a pregnancy to term* following the *birth* of one or more children. I view secondary infertility as a social and emotional crisis of infertile parents, rather than as a solely medical diagnosis. For that reason, I consider a childless woman who has conceived and miscarried to be experiencing primary infertility, whereas a woman with a child who has since repeatedly miscarried would be secondarily infertile. While a pregnancy *with the same partner* is certainly important medical data, I feel that the presence or absence of children is what shapes the emotional experience. The following account describes a typical situation:

> It was painful. All around me, my friends from my playgroup (mostly younger) and other acquaintances I had made since Joe's birth were all having their second children, seemingly without problems. This accentuated for me one of the unique problems of secondary infertility: If we had not succeeded in having a child, we would have oriented our lives differently and not surrounded ourselves with kids as much. . . . We're constantly in touch with families with two (or more) children, which creates this constant reminder of what we don't have.

Secondary infertility can and does occur among couples who earlier had little or no problem conceiving, as well as among those with a recurring infertility problem, who can be said to have experienced both primary and secondary infertility. A woman and/or her partner may have had one or more children from a previous relationship and find themselves infertile now as a couple. In this case, they would not fit neatly into any category. Nor would adoptive parents who are trying to conceive.

Unfortunately, many couples fail to recognize themselves as infertile and to seek help for secondary infertility. According to Karen Berkeley, a former staff member at the national offices of RESOLVE, Inc., a support and advocacy organization for infertile individuals, callers with children will often ask if they are eligible for services. (This issue is discussed in Chapter 5, "Caught between Two Worlds.") Some do not even contact RESOLVE, feeling that they do not fit the definition:

> As I think back on it, one of my reasons for not joining a RESOLVE group on secondary infertility was my (perhaps false) assumption that most people would not have had problems with a first pregnancy.

Similarly, women with a history of pregnancy losses may not fit the narrower definition of infertile, although they too are lacking the longed-for child:

> I don't fit the exact definition of secondary infertility . . . as being "able to achieve a pregnancy in the past but . . . unable to do so again." We have one child age four and a half. Since our son's birth, we have experienced six pregnancy losses and a great deal of physical and emotional pain.

Demographics

Secondary infertility is not as rare as it seems; the condition is even more common statistically than primary infertility. According to the National Center for Health Statistics, more than half of American women who could not conceive or carry a pregnancy to term already had at least one child.[2] Other estimates set the percentage as high as 70 percent. Carla Harkness, in *The Infertility Book: A Comprehensive Medical and Emotional Guide*, states that secondary infertility affects an estimated 1.4 million American couples and an unknown number of single women.[3]

Given these figures, it is striking how many couples with secondary infertility report that they don't know anyone else with this problem. This population is less visible than those with primary infertility for two reasons: They are often assumed to be fertile because they have a child, and they are only half as likely to seek medical help as couples who have never had a child.[4] It is hard emotionally, financially, logistically, and physically to combine infertility treatments with parenting; many parents are unable to travel to clinics or to afford the costly treatments. (This problem is discussed in Chapter 9, "Considering Possible Outcomes.")

Medical Perspective

Couples who never previously experienced fertility problems are understandably reluctant to consider that possibility. Many delay seeking treatment and, when they do, are often encouraged by doctors to "wait and see." Couples who have a history of recurring infertility, on the other hand, are more apt to seek medical attention soon after or even before attempting to conceive again.

Causes

Secondary infertility has the same causes as primary infertility, with the exception of congenital factors, such as a malformed uterus. Some conditions may develop in either partner following the birth of a child, some may result from complications experienced during labor and delivery, and some preexisting, if unidentified, problems may have worsened over time. The time interval between the prior birth and the age of both partners is also a factor. Changes in general health, infections, use of prescription medications and surgery can also impair fertility in both men and women. While many cases of infertility remain undiagnosed, such "unexplained infertility" should not be used to bolster the argument that infertility is due to stress, sexual dysfunction, or unconscious ambivalence about parenting. Stress and sexual problems may result from the infertility but are rarely the cause of it. As for emotional ambivalence, to paraphrase Barbara Eck Menning, founder of RESOLVE, Inc. "That would be the ultimate contraceptive; parents would just have to *wish* not to have more children!" Yet, you probably know other parents who did not want additional children but, ironically, still went on to have more.

Treatment/Outcome

The same treatments are available for secondary as for primary infertility. The decision of how aggressively to pursue treatment can be difficult, given today's advanced technology. There is some basis for optimism, since the rate of successful pregnancies is higher with secondary than with primary infertility. According to one medical study, "the cumulative pregnancy rate . . . for couples with a history of pregnancy in the current partnership was 56 percent, compared with 44 percent for those with primary infertility."[5] This pregnancy rate includes those who have received treatment and should not be used as a rationale to delay or forgo treatment.

The confusion and optimism that often accompany an infertility diagnosis for those who have earlier conceived easily may not only delay treatment but also delay acceptance that there may be a problem. The following account illustrates this dynamic:

> In the beginning of our treatment, I got the feeling from our various doctors that our case was a relatively easy one and that conception would be achieved. At that time, I too was optimistic. Our fertility doctor did mention that the fact that we had conceived in the past and carried a baby to term was in our favor.
>
> I think the fact that we had a son who was conceived so easily also caused me to take our infertility less seriously. . . . I think that up to more recently, somewhere deep inside I kept telling myself that I really do not belong in the category of the secondary infertile—my case always seemed less severe than those in my support group—I was going to be the one to get pregnant.

Emotional Dynamics and Need for Support

Dealing with secondary infertility shares much of the same pain as experiencing primary infertility but has unique dynamics and stresses as well. As parents experiencing infertility, you do not fit easily into any group. You may feel set apart from other parents who are going on easily to have additional children; however, as parents, you may not be readily accepted by the childless infertile.

You may have been shocked by the pain of infertility; for many, it represents a life crisis that calls for much emotional support. It is often hard for family and friends to comprehend and respond to this pain. You may have found that you and your spouse experience infertility differently from one another; couples are frequently out of sync in their reactions.

Personal Narratives

This book draws upon first-person accounts submitted in response to notices placed in the RESOLVE national newsletter and in *Stepping Stone* newsletter. Responses were received from sixty women, from twenty-five states, Canada, and Israel. The women ranged from twenty-eight to forty-six years old; the median age was thirty-six. They had children ranging from two and three-quarters to twenty-three years old. The women who sent material represent a cross-section of infertility statuses: those undergoing treatment, some who had experienced recent pregnancy losses, some with absolute diagnoses (hysterectomy), others who were pregnant or who had completed their families through birth or adoption.

All of these women identified themselves as secondarily infertile, were involved with either RESOLVE, Inc., or the Stepping Stone ministry, and felt strongly enough about this issue to write their stories and/or respond to a survey questionnaire. Their responses are not representative of all women experiencing secondary infertility, particularly the group that does not pursue treatment. Each, however, shared her own personal truth, and many common themes emerged. I hope that their stories will provide you with insight into the secondary infertility experience of others and validate your own experiences. These accounts do not illustrate a "right" or "wrong" way to respond to this crisis, nor unfortunately, do they provide easy answers as to how to get through it. Presented here rather are how various parents have dealt with being infertile and some suggestions about what has been helpful to others.

Style of Presentation

Despite the common dynamics of infertility, each couple's and each individual's stories are unique. At times, I generalize or oversimplify in order to avoid confusing qualifications and disclaimers. While few statements will hold for everyone, much of the material presented reflects common experiences and feelings.

In some cases, I have slightly edited quotations for clarity or length and assigned pseudonyms in the interests of respecting the privacy of the respondents' children. Otherwise, these are faithful representations of what was submitted, unedited for pain or anger.

Bear in mind that these vignettes are snapshots of how people felt at a given time; hopefully, many are now at a more comfortable place. Still, I wanted you to share in the highs and lows of their journeys.

As for language, all of the respondents were female, so the terms *she, her,* and *mother* are commonly used. I would like to acknowledge that infertility is a couples problem that in some cases is even more painful to a husband than to his wife. Since this is an exception to the usual pattern, women's reactions are presented to a greater extent than their partners'. Also, I am well aware that many of the secondarily infertile have two or more children; again, for clarity the term *child* is often used when *child or children* is intended. Similarly, since all of the respondents were married, the term *spouse* is often used when *partner* would be more inclusive.

Organization of the Book

In the first section of this book I focus on the social and emotional issues of secondary infertility, including symptoms such as anger and depression; the effects on the marriage; relationships with family, friends, and co-workers; and the unique isolation that accompanies secondary infertility.

Next, I examine parenting issues, such as the effect of the infertility on the child, as well as more general parenting concerns: raising a single child, spacing siblings, feeling overprotective, trying to hold on to your child, and parenting while undergoing the stresses of treatment.

In the final section I explore possible outcomes, such as adopting, continuing or ending treatment, using third parties as donors and affirming the family as is. I suggest some strategies and resources for coping which I hope will be helpful to you; however, in no way are they a substitute for medical advice, peer support, or professional counseling.

I

Social and Emotional Issues

2

The Emotional Impacts of Secondary Infertility

I just want to crawl into a cave and never come out.
—Mother following pregnancy loss

Secondary infertility hurts. You may have been surprised by how much. You probably never anticipated that the inability to complete your desired family could cause so much pain. Yet, there is no way to anticipate how you will react to the pivotal experience of becoming parents, or how central parenting can become to your sense of self and well-being.

Secondary infertility shares much of the pain of primary infertility but has other losses associated with it as well. Common reactions are denial, shock, anger, guilt, a sense of being out of control, depression, grief, and isolation. One woman describes the range of emotions she has experienced while dealing with her infertility.

What are the emotions I have felt over the years? Here goes:

1. *Shock*, initially, assuming we would have no problem conceiving.
2. *Frustration*—why didn't it just happen again?
3. *Jealousy*—of other friends so easily getting pregnant with second children.
4. *Feeling alone* in my feelings, especially when told that I should feel lucky to have just one.
5. *Guilt* over not being able to be satisfied with just one child, especially one as wonderful as ours.
6. *Depression*—when treatment . . . didn't work.

7. Finally, a certain degree of *acceptance* when it felt we were ready to move on to adoption.
8. Now a mixture of *apprehension* (what child will we get?) and extreme *impatience* (when are we going to have a child referred to us?).

Which emotions predominate may be a function of many factors: your fertility history, personal situation, and personality style. There is no one correct way to react, and emotions change over time.

Reactions to Recurring/First-Time Infertility

Just as the experience of secondary infertility differs from that of primary infertility, so too do differences exist even among those undergoing secondary infertility. You may have conceived easily the first time; some report becoming pregnant the first time they "tried," if not before. In this case, infertility probably was a shock, and you may have been tempted to deny it was happening to you.

One woman characterized her reaction as "lots of denial," explaining, "At first, I didn't really place myself in the category of infertility. I went through the work-up but really thought that at any point I would magically just become pregnant." Another reacted similarly: "My fantasy was that it wasn't really infertility." After all, you have proven your fertility. As one woman explains, "The one major thought in my mind through all of this has been, Why did [pregnancy] happen once for me but didn't happen again?"

Or perhaps you know too well about infertility. However, you may have hoped that you were no longer infertile, or, been optimistic that any problems could be solved as they had been in the past.

You may recognize some of the following reactions to the recurrence of infertility: "déjà vu—all the old feelings keep coming back"; disbelief that it is "happening again and the prognosis is not great"; and frustration, particularly if the treatment that once worked is no longer effective.

Because IUI [intrauterine insemination] had worked successfully the first time, we thought we'd solved the problem and would just do it again and have another child. Wrong!

Those with recurring infertility have different reactions from the responses of those confronting infertility for the first time. Whether or not you assume yourself to be fertile can affect your re-action:

> I was mentally prepared since my doctor told me 50 percent of patients who have trouble conceiving the first time will also have trouble with the second. Secondary was easier to handle also since I at least had *one* child. . . . I think we both [primary and secondary] experience emo-tional pain—but I think the childless infertile is *worse*. Once I had a child, the (emotional) pain was less severe. I was so thankful to have *one* child!

Others feel just as bad as they did before, or even worse, with the additional feelings of guilt that they "shouldn't be feeling these awful, jealous feelings again."

Shock

The recent focus on reproductive choice, particularly regarding fer-tility choice and the spacing of siblings, has created the belief that reproduction is a process that you can control. Often the only per-ceived problem is choosing if and when to have children and how many children to have, since it is commonly assumed that concep-tion will occur readily when desired. Such a belief may explain why the discovery of infertility is almost always a shock. The shock is even greater if you have proven your fertility and must later rede-fine your self-image to include the possibility and then the reality of infertility. Research documents that:

> A study has shown that children take it for granted that they will be fertile. So do most adults, until they find out differently. To change an image of oneself from a person who is fertile to that of one who is not is a painful process. Self-doubt has to be faced about the functioning of one's body . . . along with a feeling of shame and guilt. . . . Such experiences tend to lower one's self-esteem which is the biggest hazard of the ordeal.[1]

If you later learn that you are no longer fertile, then the prior as-sumption of fertility seems cruelly ironic. Sometimes couples blame themselves in retrospect for having taken their fertility for granted.

the change in fertility status is especially abrupt and

had a healthy beautiful girl. [Two years later,] I went to my gynecologist to get a prescription for pregnancy vitamins so I could plan for excellent prenatal care. I had ditched the diaphragm and was ready for another beautiful child. Instead, tumors were found, and [in less than a month] I had a total hysterectomy. My dream of ever having another child was gone, 100 percent gone, no hope, no chance, no possibility, no error, no margin for error, no blocked tube, no question of infertility. The choice is gone.

Similarly, women who are diagnosed with early cessation of ovarian function (premature menopause) are shocked to learn they are no longer fertile.[2]

Self-blame and Self-image

The inability to make sense of your diagnosis and the desire to find a reason for your misfortune might lead you to examine your own life in the hope that you can identify why you are being "punished" with infertility. The initial reaction to bad news of "Why me?" is for some soon followed by the answer "Of course, me." Barbara Eck Menning believes that it is logical for people to try to establish a cause-and-effect relationship for infertility.[3] The very randomness of infertility may be more frightening than linking the infertility to some past wrongdoing, real or imagined. If indeed the infertility is your "fault," then you might be able to atone and thereby regain control over the situation rather than being a helpless, if innocent, victim.

The vague feelings of "not being a good person" that Barbara Menning cites are compounded for some parents by the magical thinking that tells them they are being denied another child because they have not been good enough parents. In this case, two potentially guilt-producing experiences can converge: infertility and the normal imperfections of parenting. One mother who had a stillborn child and was then diagnosed with early cessation of ovarian function describes her attempts to understand why:

I don't know. I used to beat myself up over trying to figure out what I did to deserve this stuff. I have gotten mad at God. If children are blessings from God, why don't I deserve a blessing? . . . Wasn't I a good mother?[4]

Self-blaming attributions for fertility may seem farfetched. Yet they could also be regarded as a legacy of earlier myth and misinformation that continue to affect current attitudes and beliefs about infertility. Just as in biblical times, society still expects you to produce not only a child but also children. Traditional religious and cultural explanations of infertility tended to "blame the victim" for the problem and attributed fertility to a state of grace, equating it with divine favor. The Psalms offered praise to the Lord for enabling "the barren woman to dwell in her house as the joyful mother of children" (Psalms 113:9). Unfortunately, the corollary emerging from the belief in divine intervention is that infertility is somehow "the judgment of an angry God" and that if you are infertile, then you are not deserving or have been singled out for punishment.

It is difficult not to internalize this view and to blame yourself for causing the problem. For those experiencing secondary infertility, the most common regret, as mentioned previously, is not having had additional children earlier, while everything was "working." Some question whether they were meant to have more children or if pursing high-tech solutions is contrary to religious teachings. Following a hysterectomy, a woman reflects, "Now I am wondering if the universe/God wanted me to have only one."

Even though you may know rationally that you did not cause your infertility, sometimes prior life events seem to provide the answer:

I gave birth when I was eighteen years old and unmarried. Eight years later, I married my husband, and one and a half years later, learned that I might be infertile. . . . At this point in time, the most difficult thing to handle was that at seventeen, as a non-Christian, unmarried, I was alone and pregnant; now, at almost thirty, married, a Christian, seeking. . . . children, there were major complications. . . . Many times we questioned why I was able in all the wrong circumstances to conceive, yet unable to in all the right circumstances. . . . I felt it was my punishment.

Besides illustrating the dynamic of self-blame, the above account touches on another key theme: fairness. When you know you are a good parent, it is hard to understand why neglectful or even abusive parents are "blessed" with more children. A woman who can have no more pregnancies poses the common refrain "Why me?":

> It doesn't seem fair. I had a beautiful pregnancy. . . . I was looking forward to two more. Why does it have to be me who has to think about adoption? I know so many women who hated their pregnancies and hated giving birth. It's just not fair.[5]

Recognizing that goodness is not always rewarded and that "bad things happen to good people" is sobering and may be difficult to accept.

Even if your life seems perfect to outsiders, departing from the life script you have set for yourself can result in feelings of failure and a negative self-image:

> I conceived my first child on my honeymoon at the age of thirty-one. When my son was about twenty-two months, I conceived again the first month we tried to have a baby. . . . My husband and I started to try for a third child when I was almost thirty-seven and he was forty-five. We thought we had fertility in the bag. . . . Within a few months of trying to have a third child, I was overcome with emotions that I found very difficult to cope with. There were the feelings of grief, such as disbelief, anger, and intense sorrow. It would be some time before I realized that I was grieving for the phantom child. Added to these were overwhelming feelings of having failed. I had failed my husband in his desire to be a father again and had failed my two children in their desire for a sibling. My body failing me was the worst of all, though. Suddenly, I felt old.

Other women confirm this change in self-image, recounting feelings of defectiveness and of being old "because my insides were already too old to have another baby."

Depression

The pervasiveness of the depression that can accompany secondary infertility is underestimated not only by the general public but also by those experiencing it. Sometimes husbands lacking knowledge about the condition may worry that their wives are overreacting.

Women themselves may question why they aren't coping "better" with their frustration and disappointment, failing to realize that they are indeed grieving for the child they may not have. One woman addresses what the loss means in her own life: "Well, I feel like the two other children I had dreamed of are now dead. The loss really feels like a death, not a disappointment."

Another woman compares the often unrecognized loss of future children with the experience of her mother's death:

> I can say with all honesty that this has been the most difficult four years of my life. Even dealing with my mother's sudden death nine years ago was not as emotionally taxing. . . . I had my times of depression when it all looked so hopeless—when I would spend hours in a day crying on the couch while my husband was helpless to comfort me. My marriage suffered, and even my ability to enjoy my two young children.

The lack of understanding of the enormousness of the loss and the resulting tendency to minimize the accompanying depression may prevent you from receiving the help you need to cope with this life crisis. The following account describes what may well have been a clinical depression and one woman's attempts to cope with it:

> When I started my period after the [in vitro fertilization] cycle, I thought I wanted to die. I went into a depression so bad I needed professional help. I literally did not care about life. I don't remember what I wore, how I looked, being able to function at my job. I just didn't care. I thought of dying and wished I was old and physically sick so it wouldn't take too long. Even my little son did not bring any comfort to me. I was trying so hard to find a dream that I couldn't see reality. . . . I truly became like a walking zombie. I still got up, showered, and dressed, but I didn't remember anything. My whole life was a blur. All I talked about was how I wanted a baby. . . . I could not bear to see a pregnant woman or a small child. I would just begin crying uncontrollably. Once when I was shopping, I looked on a table and saw a little pair of infant booties. I just stared at them and felt like my stomach was punched in with a fist. I left the store in tears. It was like that for almost a year.

One symptom of clinical depression is the inability to take pleasure in activities you previously enjoyed. Many parents allude to the decreased enjoyment of childrearing. Unfortunately, you do not have the option of calling in "sick" or taking a "mental health day" off from parenting. The inability to fully enjoy your child can compound the loss; the potential effects of the infertility and parental depression on the child are discussed in Chapters 6 and 7.

Anger and Jealousy

Another loss you might experience is of the self you have known. Most people have an image of themselves as kind, understanding, generous, and caring toward others. This may be particularly true for parents, who have become accustomed to putting the needs of others before their own. It is difficult to reconcile this self-image with the normal feelings of anger and jealousy that accompany infertility. You might be distressed if you can no longer be happy for pregnant friends, and you might question what is wrong with you if you shy away from holding a friend's baby or attending baby showers. (This issue is discussed in Chapter 4.) Such reactions are a natural, self-protective impulse and serve to insulate you from pain. The reaction is to the situation and does not mean that you are any less caring than in the past; the cost of reaching out may now be greater, however. Similarly, the envy that so often arises does not mean that you have changed; evidence of others' fertility serves to highlight your own loss and is painful.

When a friend mentions unplanned pregnancies and appears to lack appreciation for your struggle, this can seem to trivialize your loss:

> Emotionally, it was a relief to give up, but about this time several friends and neighbors were experiencing their third or fourth pregnancies and more than one jokingly admitted to being surprised by the impending event. Hearing these flippant statements made me furious. It was almost impossible to feign sympathy for the morning sickness and aches and pains these women were experiencing.

It is difficult to empathize with what may be a crisis in such friends' lives: an unplanned pregnancy.

Another woman is upfront with her angry and envious feelings, but acknowledges her shame at feeling the way she does:

> I say I wouldn't wish it on my worst enemy. But that's not true. I wish it regularly, daily, upon every pregnant woman I see. I wish my infertility in exchange for her ability to be pregnant. It's almost involuntary. My rage cannot be controlled. When it seeps beyond the confines of my own mind, I feel rather ashamed of myself. It's spilling over pretty freely these days.

Anger may be the dominant emotion following a recent loss and may later be channeled into decision making about alternatives and help seeking. The following was written almost immediately after a pregnancy loss and reflects the intensity and immediacy of that loss:

> My fourth D&C was completed two days ago, and I am now at home. I don't think I will ever be able to leave my house and deal with people. I hung a "No Visitors" sign on my door, which is keeping people away for the most part. . . . It was supposed to be different this time. . . . I cry all the time and feel that I can't go on. I can't decide whether to stop trying or not. . . . I have all but lost my faith in God. . . . I hate all pregnant people. I hate people with babies—I'm bitter. . . . I just want to crawl into a cave and never come out.

Eventually, once this woman felt able to deal with people, she took the sign down, reflecting that "it helped me tremendously and gave me a small amount of control in a situation which leaves you with very little control."

Sense of Time Passing

If you are dealing with infertility, you may find yourself affected by milestones that mark the passage of time and underscore the gap between where you are and where you would like to be. Holidays, birthdays, anniversaries—all can have this effect. As parents experiencing infertility, you have an ever-present, tangible reminder of the passage of time: your child or children. Significant events in your child's life—entry into kindergarten, first communion, even crossing the street alone—may cause feelings of loss along with the pride. Every advance is particularly poignant, once you fear you will never experience this age again. (This dynamic is explored in Chapter 7.) If you have a history of infertility, this may be an ongoing concern:

Every stage that my son goes through, I wonder, Is this the last time I'll do this (being excited about first smile, first tooth, first word, first steps, last diaper changed, first day of preschool, etc.)?

I wonder if I'll ever do this again. It was hard taking away her bottle, the crib, the high chair, etc. The only easy stage to get through was potty-training.

I started a journal of all the cute things my son has said—because I know I'll never hear those innocent, babylike words and phrases again.

Ideas about appropriate family spacing (as discussed in Chapter 7) and the increasing financial needs of older children also add to the perceived sense of urgency regarding timing. One woman with recurring infertility explains her dilemma:

Our daughter is approaching college age in just another decade; we are faced with financial questions which we did not have to deal with last time. How much money should we spend on trying to have another child, money that otherwise we could be saving for her college? Should we spend $10,000 for a GIFT [gamete intrafallopian transfer] procedure which still might not work, or should we invest the money for her future?

The Emotional Impact of Being a Parent

Feelings about the infertility are closely entwined with your feelings about parenting and your child and are discussed in depth in Chapter 7. Being a parent influences not only your own, but others' reactions to the situation:

I knew what I was missing. Others weren't always sympathetic, pointing out how lucky I was to have one child. I hated the isolation. Most of all, I felt for my "only child," who wanted a sibling desperately.

In addition to sensing the passage of time, you might feel guilt or sorrow at being unable to provide your child with a sibling. If your child asks for siblings, the pain may be exacerbated. An article in the *RESOLVE of Ohio Newsletter* describes one little boy's pleas for a brother: "He asks us who his brothers are and when Mommy is going to have a baby in her tummy like his friends' mommies do. . . . When he says his nightly prayers, he asks God to give babies to Patches the cat and to Mommy."[6] One woman consulted her therapist about her son's "imaginary sister." Although she was assured that many "only" children have imaginary siblings as opposed to the more familiar imaginary friends, she reported still feeling a "pang of hurt . . . when my son goes on and on about his 'sister.'" On the other hand, having a child while going through infertility for some "makes it more bearable." Said one mother, "I can force myself to concentrate on him and his activities. I love him every minute."

Those who have experienced recurring infertility have a perspective from which to evaluate the impacts of both primary and secondary infertility on their lives. There is no consensus on which was the harder experience; the only agreement is that both are painful. For many, a crucial difference between primary and secondary infertility is the perception that secondary infertility is less recognized and, accordingly, receives less support and sympathy. Misunderstandings are frequent:

> People were saying (and still do), "Isn't it time for another one?" I mentioned to one of his preschool classmates' moms what a good child and sleeper Paul was. She said, "Well, if he's so good, how come you haven't had more?". . . . There were times that I wanted to wear a huge sign that said, "I don't have an only child by choice—I want more!"

(The issues unique to secondary infertility are discussed in Chapter 5, "Caught between Two Worlds.")

Resolving the Emotional Impacts

Just as the woman cited earlier removed the "No Visitors" sign once she had regained some degree of control, so will you gain perspective on your loss and gradually resolve your feelings. You may need to grieve for the fantasized family that you may be unable to have before you are able to refocus on choosing alternative outcomes, as is discussed in Section III. The following account shows one woman's progression toward acceptance of the infertility:

> Sometimes, many times, I feel so very alone with this heartache. Few people realize the magnitude with which this affects me. There are

times when I feel like I cannot stop crying, that this is the worst afflic-
tion God could hit me with, and that this pain and yearning will be
with me until the day I die. I used to pray daily that God would help us
to become pregnant. Now I pray that I will learn to accept this. That I
will be able to hear someone's excited voice telling me they're pregnant
without feeling like my guts are being wrenched out of me. I want to be
able to witness someone's protruding belly without having a wave of
envy wash over me—leaving me feeling empty and inadequate. I want
to stop counting the days of my cycle, wondering if I've ovulated and
hoping that I'm pregnant.

For this woman, a desire for an end to the emotional upheaval of
the infertility has taken precedence over even her desire for a pregnancy. You should bear in mind that there are no shortcuts to resolving the pain that accompanies infertility. (Coping strategies are
presented in chapter 10.) You must acknowledge and deal with the
emotions in order to transcend them. Although most people move
beyond their infertility, you may not leave it behind you entirely. It
can remain a part of your life experience, and for some an echo of
the old feelings remains. As Menning quotes,

My infertility resides in my heart as an old friend. I do not hear from it
for weeks at a time, and then, a moment, a thought, a baby announcement or some such thing, and I will feel the tug—maybe even be sad or
shed a few tears. And I think, "There's my old friend." It will always be
a part of me.[7]

3

Weathering Secondary Infertility as a Couple

My husband just didn't understand. . . .
—Woman experiencing secondary infertility

Infertility can challenge even the best marriage. The problem affects you both, but usually in different ways. You are both under stress, and yet are called upon to support one another, often without the support of others. Even though you may be closely allied in the struggle against infertility, you are also natural targets for one another's anger.

Further, you each bring your own coping mechanisms and personal expectations to the resolution of a shared problem. Differing sexual frames of reference and some gender-linked ways of handling emotions often make it hard for husbands and wives to empathize with one another. Frequently couples are out of sync, with one partner wanting to confront the problem just as the other needs to take a break.

Infertility is often a long-standing problem; you may be able to rally for an immediate, short-term crisis, but find the day-in, day-out strain of long-term infertility difficult to endure. Reactions to the infertility and to one another may change over time:

> At first, I think adversity pulled us together. But he was ready to quit *long* before I was. Then it became divisive. It has changed our relationship forever—some good, some bad. We are still rebuilding.

Another woman with recurring infertility conveys the difference in her experience the second time around: "The first time, it made us very close. This time, I was more reluctant to burden him and leaned more on friends."

The fact that the infertility struggle can last so long may also mean that the marriage has been on hold and that you have been unable to focus on your relationship as a priority. One wife explains:

> It is easy to lose perspective and put all our time and effort into conceiving another child and not concentrating on being a good parent or spouse. It is very hard on a marriage to be infertile. It is frustrating and emotionally exhausting.

Not only may you have been neglecting your relationship, but also you are subject to the long-term stress caused by "depleting emotional and financial reserves."

Unique Dynamics of Secondary Infertility

While some of these stresses exist in couples whether or not they are already parents, couples experiencing secondary infertility have additional issues to deal with. The pressure of parenting is an added stress; however, as parents you may also have an increased commitment to your family and to maintaining the marriage, a commitment that in turn provides motivation to work through the current stresses. For example, one woman recounts fights with her husband over whether or not they would try again and describes their relationship as "shaky," but says that were it not for their daughter, she would have "packed [her] bags and left long ago." Hopefully, sticking it out enabled this couple to resolve some of their problems.

Couples experiencing secondary infertility appear to be further apart from one another in their feelings on the issue than those with no children. Childless women express more feelings of guilt at not "giving" their husbands children; on the other hand, both partners are more apt to share the goal of having a child. In contrast, many secondarily infertile women feel that their partners are not as invested as they are in having another child.

Because you are parents already, you may experience some normal ambivalence about having additional children. Since for many couples the decision to increase a family is less clear-cut than whether to have children at all, you and your partner may find yourselves holding varying positions. Some men may be satisfied with one child; others, while they might prefer more children, can see advantages to the status quo. As one respondent indicates, "My husband was more 50–50 about having a second child; he says this is a financial thing, and if we had more money, he'd be more inclined to want a second one." Knowledge of the demands of parenting can make either parent more hesitant; however, knowing its fulfillments can also serve to eliminate any prior ambivalence.

The desire to perpetuate the parenting role is generally more characteristic of mothers than fathers. (See Chapter 7.) Traditionally, mothering has been the primary source of gratification for women, while for men parenting is one of multiple roles. Interestingly, women who also work outside the home still seem more invested in the parenting role than their male counterparts do. Fathers tend to be more pragmatic about parenthood, while it remains a central, cherished role for many women. One woman compares her reaction to her husband's:

> I have wanted this second child much more than Dan. He has been aware of how much easier our life has gotten now that our son is older and asked, "Why do you want to complicate things again?"

Most fertile couples overcome any ambivalence and readily adapt to the arrival of an additional child, even when the event was unplanned. Secondary infertility requires you to make a conscious, joint decision to pursue either treatment or adoption. The discussion about whether or not to adopt can polarize you and your spouse. Often the woman feels a compelling need for another child, while her husband is either content with the family as is or even actively opposed to adoption.

Gender Differences

While women may feel the emotional strains of infertility, their husbands focus more on the financial strains of treatment and/or adoption. Their different priorities exacerbate the tensions surrounding decision-making, sometimes to the point of needing a third party to mediate. One woman describes the need for and benefits of counseling:

[Concerning adoption,] my husband and I were at opposite ends of the continuum. I would have sold our house to get the money, but he was content with our family as it was and was urging me to consider the same. . . .

We began to see a counselor because our relationship seemed to be deteriorating. I felt that my husband just didn't understand what I was experiencing. The infertility problems seemed to be coming out in all aspects of our marriage. Counseling was very helpful.

Men have their own issues that are exacerbated by the infertility. While their sense of self may not be as tied in with the parenting role, they may be very invested in taking care of their families. This sense of responsibility can cause feelings of failure if they feel that they are unequal to the task and that they can no longer make their wives happy. Traditionally, men have defined themselves in the provider role, just as women have defined themselves as nurturers. Even when both spouses are employed, the man often feels primarily responsible for providing financial support. Miriam Mazor, M.D., an adult and child psychiatrist, feels that men need to be given permission to express what they and others may consider unacceptable feelings. She has seen much ambivalence among male patients experiencing secondary infertility, which she in part attributes to their concerns about providing for another child, particularly due to a poor economy and their advanced paternal age. In addition to the expenses of infertility and/or adoption, they may worry about saving for retirement and college expenses. If his wife desperately wants another child, a husband may be ashamed of his ambivalence and feel bad that he cannot provide unlimited financial resources. It is important that the husband's feelings be legitimized, listened to, and addressed.

Overwhelmingly, the women surveyed for this book perceive that they experience more grief than their husbands at the prospect of not having additional children. One woman epitomizes the distinction by describing her reactions as "much 'rawer,' quicker, deeper, and more often expressed." Across the board, men are depicted by their wives as less emotional about the infertility. Men are typically described as being "not one to get upset" or "more philosophical about it," while women characterize themselves as being "an emotional wreck" or "a basketcase." This is consistent with my earlier research, which showed that women are significantly more angry and depressed by infertility than their male counterparts.[1]

Repeatedly, women allege that the hardest part of the infertility for their spouses has been "putting up with" them. Husbands are also seen as vicariously experiencing their wives' pain more often than as dealing with their own. It is difficult to determine whether men are actually less emotional or are merely reluctant to share their feelings with their spouses. Some husbands fear that their own distress will make their wives feel worse, believe that emotional responses are "unmanly," or simply are not in touch with their feelings around this issue. Others feel that since they are not undergoing all the medical interventions, they are not entitled to feel as bad. One woman speculates about what her husband "really feels":

> I think that secondary infertility may be experienced differently by women and their spouses—no kidding, Sherlock! Right after we were married, my husband talked of having three kids and how it would be great to have them close together. . . . Now, however, when I try to explain my frustration at not conceiving and my fear that I won't ever have a second child, my husband tries to make me feel better by telling me that one child is really OK. . . . I wish that he could say that it is a disappointment to him and that he really wants more kids too. Maybe this is the old "male and female"—discuss what you *really* feel—dilemma.

While women's stronger responses are well documented, increasingly there is hard evidence that men too are distressed by infertility.[2] Half of the men in my study of RESOLVE members admitted to experiencing depression about the infertility. The number might have been even higher had I used a less clinical term.[3]

Typically, couples are somewhat out of sync in their reactions. Often women take the lead in dealing with the infertility. It seems that many men are optimistic at first that things will work out, while their wives are quicker to despair. One woman recounts such a time lag:

> It took him a while to catch up to me. He kept thinking it would happen for the first eighteen months or so. After that, we felt similarly sad about it, although we didn't necessarily feel the same things at the same time.

Research confirms the existence of a time lag, with men retaining their hopefulness for up to three years before addressing the potential loss.[4]

While a woman may mourn the potential loss of future children, her husband may grieve for the more immediate loss of his wife who he feels has changed. Even husbands who try to be supportive get upset with their wives for being depressed: "He doesn't know what to do with a wife who cries all the time"; "He feels I'm not always thankful for what I have." Some men feel threatened by their wives' "obsession" with the infertility, feeling that they are less important, or they may feel jealous that their wives are too depleted to give them the attention they want. It is difficult to admit these needy feelings; anger at the infertility or at their wives' reactions may be easier and more acceptable responses for some men.

Some men feel that their wives are fixated more on what they don't have than on what they do have. One woman ruefully compares her existing relationship with her husband with her longing for a desired child:

> I feel it would be easy for me to find another husband. It's nearly impossible to "find" another child.

Such a husband might feel devalued if the reaction cited above were taken literally, rather than as reflecting temporary despair.

Some losses are linked to gender, and a partner can only try to empathize with the other's pain:

> It has something to do with identity for me more than him, I think. This is probably a difference in men and women, but I always have known that I wanted to be a mother, so it goes back further for me.

Additionally, the desire to recapture the experiences of pregnancy, childbirth, and nursing occasions strong feelings in many women. The following vignette describes a loss only a mother can experience:

> For me, the greatest difficulty is giving up the pregnancy I may never have [again]. A few weeks ago, I was shopping in a large indoor mall in Chicago and passed by a store which specialized in maternity clothing for professional women. I found that I couldn't even look at the beautiful outfits draped on the pregnant mannequins. The sense of loss was

just overwhelming, and I thought, I might never be able to wear maternity clothes again.

In the above quotation, for this woman the maternity clothes seem to represent the loss of the longed-for pregnancy and the chance to mother an infant again.

Infertility can affect how you feel about your body and your sense of self. The perception that your body is no longer performing its function can lead to feelings of inadequacy and even failure. The fact that most often the woman undergoes treatment contributes to the varying impact of the total experience:

My husband does not have to live with infertility daily. He does not suffer the side effects of fertility drugs or lay in bed with a thermometer, unable to get up while my toddler cries to get out of her crib. He does not wonder at the end of each month if the cramps really mean we failed again. He can forget a lot easier.

It is difficult for men to empathize with the disappointment at the onset of menstruation and the intrusiveness of some of the procedures, just as women do not fully comprehend how their husbands feel about sex on demand or producing semen specimens. Physical differences account for some of the dissimilar feelings about the infertility, as one woman explains:

My partner is more removed from the reminders. Physically, I am very attuned to my body's signs of ovulation and menstruation. It is difficult to turn this off when I've been watching these signs through years of infertility. These signs remind me throughout every month that it has not happened . . . again. He also is occupied with work and non-baby-related activities for most of his day. This makes it easier for him to forget.

As this implies, women are also more often on the front lines, dealing with pregnant women and seeing babies. This is the case both at home and at work; pregnant women and new mothers populate the office as well as the playground. Further, women are apt to feel isolated from other women whose focus is on pregnancy and parenting. In general, women's lives are more closely linked to their role as parents than men's lives are. Men are less likely to discuss details of pregnancies or childrearing.

Impact of the Diagnosis

In some instances, the partner who is assumed to be fertile may feel the need to repress his or her own feelings so as not to seem to be "blaming" the spouse, while the spouse with the identified problem may feel guilty and vulnerable and even offer to end the relationship. In the majority of cases, the infertility is attributable to either male or female factors in about equal numbers (about 40% for each). A smaller group exists in which both partners contribute to the infertility. Such differences in fertility status can create a barrier to sharing mutual feelings about a problem that affects you both regardless of the diagnosis.

When the difficulty is identified as a male factor, certain issues commonly arise. Men tend not to share their diagnosis with others. Their wives may feel set apart from infertile women because the problem is not within their own bodies, while they must share with their husbands the frustration of infertility treatments such as intrauterine insemination or even IVF, aimed at compensating for their husbands' problem. Because donor insemination is a possibility and they may be considering secrecy, some couples can't discuss their problem with others. Men are understandably shocked to learn of a male factor, particularly after having fathered a child:

> He definitely was shocked when we learned of his low sperm count, but it didn't take him long to accept it. He is easily distracted by his work and school and raising our daughter. If it was up to him, we would stop all medical interventions and just let nature take its course, even if that means not having a second child.

In this case, the wife felt resentful for being "the one carrying it around with me all day and night" until her husband agreed to try donor insemination. (Third party reproductive options are discussed in Chapter 9.)

Men are affected by the knowledge that they have an infertility problem. A woman relates her husband's grief in not being able to give her "the one thing I desperately wanted from him." One husband whose wife described him as "also very distraught" was said to be "carrying the weight of the responsibility." Yet even in this case, his wife still thinks the infertility has been "more physically and emotionally crippling" for her.

Effect on the Marital Relationship

Any loss or crisis has the potential not only to create strain in your marriage but also to deepen the bond. For most crises, you may have a natural support network of family and friends that you can call upon. But infertility can be isolating, causing you to depend almost entirely on one another. In some cases, the isolation serves to draw you closer to one another. The following describes this positive outcome:

> In a strange way, we are actually closer, because we are the only ones who really understand the other. I can be honest with him when I feel I can't be brutally honest with anyone else.

Some report that the need to rely on one another has led them to perceive each other as "best friends." One woman credits her husband, who let her talk for hours, as being a "tremendous part of [her] healing." As another woman put it, she and her husband have become "closer for all the up and downs (mainly downs)."

Most likely, you will cope as you have in other crises; the knowledge that you have survived rough times in the past can be a source of reassurance. One woman relates that while she and her partner

> in no way sailed through last couple of years, . . . we came to deal with all the issues of the infertility treatments and ups and downs pretty much like we've coped with our other challenges of married life. . . . We struggled, argued, cried, reassured, and ultimately worked through it all. . . . Yes, we've been affected by infertility, but our marriage bond has not been threatened by it all.

Some of you may have outside resources you have used in the past, such as individual or couples therapists, to help navigate the current crisis. You may be aware of your reactions to loss and have developed techniques to negotiate differences and to communicate with one another. For others of you, infertility represents the first crisis of your marriage and may set the pattern for subsequent problem solving.

Being in different places emotionally and having different coping styles can create distance and a sense of estrangement between you and your spouse. This is especially true if you blame each other for not sharing feelings and think your spouse is either "indifferent" or "obsessed." In my work with couples, these terms come up repeatedly, with husbands often being more affected by their wives' reaction to the infertility than by the infertility itself. In one such couple with *"very* different reactions," according to the wife, therapy helped them to accept each other's feelings following a period in which she felt very *"separate"* from him and alone in her quest for a second child. Other husbands tire of hearing the usual but perhaps seemingly endless complaints about treatment:

> Has the relationship I have with my husband been challenged by this? Of course! Sometimes we are very united in the struggle. Sometimes I want to leave him and marry a widower with four children, because he is so uninterested in my latest medical information. If I drag my feet over another surgery or shot, he gets short-tempered and says, "Well, if you don't want a baby, don't do it," like he's tired of hearing me whine.

Sometimes women who have longed to have their husbands share their feelings are shaken when it happens, and they too experience sadness. Some couples are able to support one another by "tak[ing] turns being upset: When he is down, I find that I am strong for him and vice versa." While you may wish you shared the same feelings, you may come to realize that it is not always realistic or even desirable to feel the same way at the same time. Rather than expecting or demanding that your spouse mirror your own reactions, it is important to validate and respect each other's feelings.

Other potential sources of blame are decisions you made earlier in the relationship: to delay marriage, to use contraception, to terminate an unplanned pregnancy, and/or to postpone having more children. For example, one woman realizes that she blames her husband for recommending that she use an IUD, which led to infection and infertility. While rationally she knows that he did not want this to happen and was not responsible, it is still hard for her to dismiss the anger. If you recognize the root of any lingering anger and examine it, hopefully, you can then put it aside.

You may fear, as many couples do, that infertility will be the last straw, jeopardizing your relationship and underscoring basic and perhaps irreconcilable differences between you. Usually this is not the case. Even the following pessimistic account is not without hope that once the couple are beyond the crisis, or receive help coping, their relationship will endure:

I don't think my husband understands the depths of my despair. . . . Although I would like to say all these experiences have made my marriage stronger, I can't. My husband and I fight most in times of crisis. We deal with things very differently and don't really understand one another. He's very logical, unemotional, and accepting. So we won't have another child. . . . I doubt my marriage will [survive].

Most commonly, infertility presents a temporary crisis that you and your spouse will transcend and resolve. Even though she characterizes her husband as having "been supportive every month I get my period," one woman details the pervasive effects on their relationship:

I withdrew. I cried a lot. I didn't want to have sex. . . . It's getting better now. [But] even this summer, we went alone on a vacation and I could hardly talk to him without crying. [Still,] it's better now, as I come to accept that infertility is forever.

Effect on the Sexual Relationship

The impact of infertility on your sexual relationship presents another unexpected challenge. Both men and women report a lessened sex drive and a feeling of why "bother" with sex if they don't "have to." It is difficult for a sexual relationship to withstand the pressure of tests and routinized sex on demand. "Forced sex" has been likened to forcing someone to eat chocolate daily whether the person wants to or not, with comparable effects on the appetite for both chocolate and sex.[5] Sexual intimacy, which may have been an important part of your relationship, may instead become for some of you primarily a means for procreation: "The thought of sex totally puts me off. I only wanted to have sex when I thought I was ovulating and lost interest toward the end of my cycle."

Some couples, out of religious convictions, question whether they are entitled to enjoy sex if it cannot lead to conception. Others experience guilt or shame over prior sexual experiences or even fantasies. Further, rather than being associated with love and pleasure, sex often becomes a reminder of failure and pain: "Our marriage was terrible. I couldn't bear the thought of a sexual contact, because it would leave me crying long into the night."

While reported feelings of revulsion about making love represent an extreme reaction, you are likely to find that your sex lives are affected to some extent, at least temporarily. Acknowledging the difference is one way to take the pressure off; it is draining to try to pretend everything is the same. Identifying the degree to which infertility treatment is interfering with your sexual sharing can prevent misunderstandings and keep you from falsely attributing the decrease in sex to a decrease in caring. Also, you must realize that the problem is time-limited and does not mean that you can never regain your prior level of sexual functioning.

The idea of working to preserve a sexual relationship may seem futile to couples absorbed with parenting. Parents often have difficulty maintaining their sex lives without the added burden and stresses of infertility treatment. Sex on schedule in a home with a young child raises logistical and privacy issues. It is not unusual for postcoital tests to be canceled. Parents who share a family bed with their child report that this further complicates the situation.

You may be less able to follow the prescribed advice for sexual problems, such as planning a romantic getaway, although some parents do make arrangements to do just that. Similarly, it is hard to have spontaneous sexual relations during the nonfertile time of the month or to try new settings to separate recreational from procreational intercourse. Overall, you should try to maintain a couple identity distinct from parenting roles and to negotiate a sexual relationship at a level that respects the needs and feelings of both of you.[6]

Suggestions for Weathering Infertility as a Couple

You may find that you not only lack the child you desire to complete your family but at times feel you have lost enjoyment of your life together. On the other hand, you may experience, as some couples do, a heightened appreciation of what you do have and make a deliberate attempt to cherish each day with each other and your child.

Understanding the impact infertility can have on your relationship may help to keep problems in perspective. Realizing that your reactions are not unusual may also reduce the pressure. Knowing that the side effects of infertility, such as depression and anger, are temporary and normal may make it easier for you to accept these distressing changes. RESOLVE meetings and couples support groups, if they are available in your area, are a wonderful source of support and validation; relief spreads throughout the group when someone admits to a problem that the others have experienced but were reluctant to discuss.

Some guidelines may be helpful for negotiating this crisis. First, it is important for you to check out what your partner is really feeling rather than assuming that you know. For example, a husband may assume that his wife is angry with him when she is instead angry at the situation. Simply asking your spouse if he or she is angry and, if so, why can sometimes clarify the problem, avoid unnecessarily hurt feelings, and/or pinpoint what needs to be done in the future. It is important not to try to label what your spouse is feeling (e.g., "You don't care"), but rather to elicit his or her feelings. Conversely, stating your own feelings ("I feel alone with this problem sometimes") is less likely to elicit a defensive response than accusing your spouse of emotional abandonment.

Merle Bombardieri, a well known infertility therapist, has popularized a technique described as the "twenty-minute rule." This exercise sets a time limit on infertility discussions, thereby accomplishing dual goals: guaranteeing the spouse who is reluctant to discuss these issues that the discussions will end and assuring the partner who wishes to talk that the conversation will take place. Participation in couples support groups and/or couples therapy accomplishes the same goal of having a time and place to deal with the issue. Hiring a babysitter to get special time and space to talk about it can be effective as well.

You may need to schedule time off from your infertility. You may get so caught up in the momentum of treatment you forget that to some extent you can determine the pacing and take a vacation from treatment if you both want to. Couples who are between treatment cycles often report that this break provides an opportunity to get back in touch with themselves and each other. It is easy to underestimate the cumulative effects of months of invasive medical procedures, disappointment, and hormone treatment. Some men report that their wives are different people when taking hormones; one said that he never knew "who would be waiting for [him]" when he got home from work, even if he called ahead, because his wife's mood swings were so rapid. Couples often become somewhat matter-of-fact about incredibly arduous interventions, and the extraordinary quickly becomes commonplace. Recognizing and making allowances for the toll of treatment and taking a break when needed are ways to regain control of your lives and relationship.

Another potential source of conflict is who is responsible for the work of infertility: the treatment, the scheduling, the research into medical conditions and resources, and even the grieving. Commonly, one partner seems to take on most of these tasks and may come to resent it. Planning together for a more equitable division of labor can alleviate one source of tension. Since it is usually the woman who must undergo treatment, some men make it a point not only to go to appointments but also to contact the doctor with questions or argue with the insurance company when necessary. Giving his wife the medication injections may make a husband feel more actively involved in the process. The sense of functioning as a team, even if one partner's participation may be mainly symbolic, creates a climate of mutual support and minimizes resentment.

Another pitfall that may in part result from gender differences is the tendency for one partner (usually the husband) to try to make everything all right. While this may appear to be a desirable goal, sometimes "fixing it" is not possible, and what is really needed is empathy. Tolerating the pain of a loved one is difficult, and the impulse may be to deny the situation or to try to come up with a solution. You may be surprised to learn what your spouse really wants from you in the way of comfort. An acknowledgment of the pain or simply a hug may sometimes be enough, and better than reassurance or a rational response to the problem that does not address the emotions attached.

Michael Carter, coauthor of *Sweet Grapes: How to Stop Being Infertile and Start Living Again*, seems to speak for many men as he describes the process by which he learned to stop trying to "fix it" and instead began to successfully communicate with his wife:

> It took me a long time to learn that I really wasn't helping. Both of my strategies—silence and problem solving—were actually ways of keeping problems at arm's length. At that distance, I didn't have to feel them. I didn't have to be a part of the hurt and confusion that come with tough issues. . . .
>
> Communication grows out of the confusion and conflict within yourself or between yourself and another, and communication thrives on those differences. Confusion and disagreement are good when they

lead to communication, and communication leads to strength and understanding. . . .

I learned that you don't have to know the answers before you open your mouth and that there is no shame in not having all the answers. . . . And I learned that though problem solving is appropriate some of the time, other occasions require me to feel it, not to fix it. That sounds very feminine, doesn't it? But feeling is often much tougher than fixing, and usually far more helpful.[7]

4

Your Relationships with Family, Friends, and Co-workers

It's an incredibly lonely place.
—Woman describing the experience of secondary infertility

Secondary infertility affects not just you and your partner and child but also your parents, other relatives, friends, and work associates. The impact ranges from a teacher who finds it difficult to deal with her students' pregnant mothers to an at-home mother who plans outings based on where she will be least likely to encounter large families. It is common for women to avoid friends who are pregnant, to decline invitations to baby showers, and to put their career on hold while they are in infertility limbo. Unfortunately, infertility can strain all of your relationships.

Absence of Support

While family and friends may usually be your first source of support during illness or loss, secondary infertility is an unfamiliar and unrecognized loss and consequently is often unsupported. Infertility is invisible, and there is no concrete loss to mourn. Secondary infertility is particularly unacknowledged. Pregnancy loss, while more tangible, is still perceived as a "taboo subject," eliciting neither "standard religious customs or ceremonies" nor other forms of "societal support and comfort."[1] Since even a visible medical event such as a miscarriage may not prompt the caring that is so badly needed, it is unsurprising but nonetheless disappointing if your close friends and family fail to provide solace for your intangible recurring losses of infertility.

Both anecdotal and statistical evidence indicates that this, unfortunately, is often the case. A study of RESOLVE members found that while 80 percent of individuals felt they had received "much support" from their partner, less than one-third reported receiving "much support" from family and friends.[2] While it is desirable that you and your spouse support one another, the lack of other support can overly stress your relationship. Moreover, the lack of expected support from others can lead to disillusionment with the quality of those relationships and even estrangement from family and friends just when you most need a support network.

You may find that there is little sympathy for your problem and be frustrated by a lack of understanding from people who have not experienced infertility firsthand. (See Chapter 5, "Caught between Two Worlds," for a discussion of this uniquely isolated status.) Secondarily infertile individuals report a range of responses from their relatives: not wanting to know what's going on, not believing anyone would go through so much to have a baby, thinking it is "crazy to want more" or that the infertile relative is "joking." Other couples do not tell their families or friends about the infertility problem, thus eliminating the possibility of support from them.

Some who have experienced recurring infertility remark on the lesser degree of support they received the second time around: "People are more indifferent because I have children. People were more encouraging . . . the first time around. . . . There was more interaction." Regrettably, if others in your family are involuntarily childless, secondary infertility might be given less sympathy, since family members might consider you lucky to have a child at all. While this might seem fair and logical to them, such prioritizing hurts when you are experiencing the loss of your desired family.

Being disappointed in the response of those closest to you can exacerbate the pain. A couple learned two days before Thanksgiving that they could never conceive again, a diagnosis they shared with their family. While the couple didn't want their sadness to ruin a joyful occasion, they expected their recent bad news to be addressed:

We spent Thanksgiving with family, and our grief went unmentioned. Instead, we felt inundated with everybody talking about all the things they were thankful for, and our pain was not given any acknowledgment. . . . That was exceptionally painful to deal with, as it felt as if we were not an important part of the family.

In another scenario, the desire to have another child is not only ignored but discouraged by family members who fail to understand the feelings involved:

> I felt a great deal of pressure from family unable to understand why I would put my life on hold for this. I was told by my mother that I should stop planning my life around this drug treatment. I was told that I should just be grateful for the child I have and forget about having another. It is painful to feel that my family does not understand that I am grateful for my daughter, but I also would love to have another child.

Others actively oppose intervention, sometimes for religious reasons, and blame the individual for pursuing treatment:

> I was . . . told by some family members that what I was doing was unethical from a moral standpoint, and that it was unethical to allow my insurance to pay for these procedures. People like me were making the insurance premiums of everybody go up just because I wanted another baby, . . . a [condition] that was non-life-threatening.

While such procedures may be considered "elective" by health economists, they do not feel elective if you are trying to having another child. You don't need to hear these reservations voiced by people you want to be more concerned with your needs than with global issues of insurance coverage.

Sometimes the role you have played within your family or social group may stand in the way of your receiving support: If you have helped others, you may expect them to be there for you in turn. It is disappointing and seems unfair when your caretaking is not reciprocated. If you have never been seen as needy, it might be hard for others to recognize that you too have problems and need support. It can be a blow to your self-esteem to shed the role of the "together" one and let others know you are vulnerable. Further, there is the fear of being let down if others fail to respond. While there is no guarantee of how others will respond if they know your situation, if they don't know, not only is there no chance of receiving support but there is no way to avoid unknowing hurtful remarks.

For example, when one set of grandparents learned of their child's infertility, the grandparents were distraught over their unknowing, unnecessary, and painful admonitions for the couple to give them more grandchildren.

Seeking Support

Infertility is understandably hard to discuss. As one woman explains, "No one knows, and there is never the right time to bring it up—it's personal; I don't like sharing it with everyone." She goes on to relate a particularly painful social episode triggered by a joking exchange, an episode that seems inevitable unless those present were aware of her sensitivity to this issue.

> We went to a Christmas party last month—the big talk of the night was that twelve women in my neighborhood are pregnant, two with twins. "It must be in the water!" says everyone. I wanted to shout, "It's not in my—water!"

When you receive validation, support, or consideration after sharing your feelings, you are encouraged to share again. Confidences that are met with indifference or even insensitive remarks are understandably less likely to be repeated. It is important to bear in mind, as the following respondent points out, that people rarely mean to be unkind, but rather don't understand what may be painfully obvious to those experiencing infertility:

> Most friends and family members have responded in what they believe to be a supportive way. Most have shown concern, although unfortunately, many and most reactions and comments illustrate a basic lack of understanding of infertility and the emotions it entails. I try not to be critical of many painful and outright stupid comments, for I do realize that I too was ignorant prior to my initiation into the ranks of the infertile.

Often the people who are hurting feel the need to educate family and friends as to what is an appropriate response. This process can be draining but may be worthwhile to preserve a valued relationship. One woman characterizes her relationship with her friends by saying, "I'm constantly teaching." Whether you can take on the demanding role of a consciousness-raiser may depend on where you are in the infertility process. As one woman explains,

For the most part, people don't understand the pain and sadness of not being able to have a second child. . . . So I've discussed it very little. Maybe now that I'm feeling less raw, I might be able to help people understand. They say dumb things that hurt—unintentionally.

Sometimes partners disagree over who should be told or how much information should be shared. It is difficult if one partner wants to tell others but the other partner prefers secrecy. Some people elect to keep a zone of privacy at work, not wanting to seem vulnerable or have their commitment to the job questioned. Yet often someone at work must know, in order to allow time off for treatment.

You may fear that if you tell others, you will be plagued with inquiries at times when you prefer not to deal with the issue. Sometimes, however, a sympathetic sibling or co-worker takes on the task of educating and sensitizing others. It is also helpful to have someone who can privately alert you to potentially difficult situations: a pregnancy announcement, the visit of a co-worker's baby, etc.

We all, consciously or not, select others to confide in. Sometimes those who are usually empathetic are at a loss when confronted with infertility. You must judge who you think will be most supportive. While some describe their family as their "main untiring support, [while] friends [are] not so understanding," in other cases friends can empathize when family members do not:

Friends were *very* supportive. Female family members were NOT: They could not understand what I was going through; they get pregnant easily; they avoided me and didn't want to discuss it with me. This hurts.

Those who experienced prior infertility respond to earlier reactions:

The first time, our parents always seemed to say the wrong thing. . . . We did not tell family members we were trying again, which did eliminate some stress. The first time, we pretended to friends [that] having children was a future thought—it was difficult to live with this pretense. This time, we were open with friends, and the support was overwhelming.

How and who to tell within the family, a group of friends, or co-workers are, of course, very personal decisions.

You may be pleasantly surprised to find responsiveness from those who were never there for you before, even if you are disappointed in others. For instance:

> It takes such a crisis to really learn some things about your friendships. The friend from whom I expected the most support gave me none. Even after confronting her with how I felt, and how I wanted her to ask me how things were going, she never did, and she still does not. I was very hurt by this, and I believe it has caused some scars in our relationship. At this point, our friendship is healing, but I view it in a much different way than I did before the crisis, and I have come to the conclusion that she, as well as many others, just is not capable of understanding this type of crisis.
>
> The support that I received from other friends came from people that I never expected to provide support, and I have fostered some new and very deep and personal friendships for which I will be forever grateful. Some of these friendships came from a support group I joined, which consisted of people going through secondary infertility. These people could relate completely to my pain.

Others who have experienced loss and hardship may be best able to empathize:

> I have had positive and negative [reactions]. Some, in trying to be supportive, actually made me feel worse. However, most people were indifferent. One lady that was very supportive surprised me, since her husband was dying of cancer. I would have thought infertility would have seemed trivial to her.

Sometimes people receive support in one way from someone who is unable to support them totally, as illustrated below:

> My mother was the only one who really tried to provide support. She came from out of town to help watch my son during one of the IVF procedures. She was there physically for me, but was unable to understand my emotional rollercoaster.

Other times the support is expressed in a way that may be alienating. The following account shows how a woman was able to read between the lines and accept the caring that was intended despite the words used to convey it:

I have had a range of responses, from the typical subtle blaming (e.g., "You know, it might be that you're trying too hard," or "Your emotions may be the problem") to very empathic and understanding.

I do get the comment "Well, at least you have one." Sometimes it hurts, and sometimes it doesn't. It depends on who says it, how they say it, and how I'm feeling. Because I agree to a certain extent. It can mean "You have nothing to complain about," or it can mean "I'm so glad for you that you at least have one."

Discussing Treatment with Others

In some families, differing feelings about treatment options may lead the couple to prefer secrecy or to be selective about what they share. Some parents of secondarily infertile women are nervous about medical interventions and worried about the toll on their daughter's health:

> My mother openly asked me why I kept going through pregnancies and miscarriages, and she urged me to stop doing this to my body. But my father just told me how much he loved me and that he would support me no matter what I decided to do. Of the two, my father was more comforting.[3]

Other parents reject treatment options for religious reasons, believing that fertility is "God's will." In most families, not only is there a generation gap with respect to understanding and accepting the technologies—reproductive technology has been revolutionized in the past generation and takes much getting used to—but there may be an informational gap as well if your parents have no understanding of infertility:

> My mother, in particular (who has nine children), was so puzzled. She kept telling me stories of couples who adopted and then got pregnant. It was as though she didn't believe me. It made me irritated with her, and I felt hurt that she wasn't able to give me the kind of support I was looking for. However, over time her attitude has changed as so much time has gone by with no pregnancy, and as I fill her in about the procedures, etc., she has become more knowledgeable about infertility.

Friends too may have mixed feelings about reproductive technology. Some couples reason that they do not owe anyone else the details about their treatments, particularly if these will create unwelcome controversy.

Coping with Others' Pregnancies

Those who are in the same generation and roughly the same age may be more familiar with the technology but create different problems. They are most likely having their own families. What may once have been a shared bond now becomes a constant reminder of loss. Many couples, friends and relatives alike, become close when their first children are born. When they go on to have additional children, you may have a sense of having been left behind.

Being told about yet another pregnancy within your family or social circle is hard, but not being told can be harder still. It is often difficult for the pregnant person to share the news, knowing that it may cause you pain. Some delay sharing the news or give the task to another. Although this may be kindly meant, such special treatment may seem to be a criticism of your ability to cope and make you feel even more set apart.

Specific techniques can facilitate communication around pregnancies; you might find it easier to express your ambivalence in a note. Think about how you would like to be told about a pregnancy or birth and suggest, for example, that someone else inform you so that you are not put on the spot, but can respond when you are able. Such strategies can prevent awkward situations and rifts from occurring. One woman describes how she reacted to a close friend's pregnancy:

> Around her seventh month, I wrote her a letter explaining how difficult it was for me to deal with her and her pregnancy. Writing the letter was very therapeutic for me, and it broke the ice for us to start communicating again at a level that was emotionally comfortable for me.

You may find it easier if a friend is having her first child rather than a second or third child. Some women have an easier time accepting a friend's subsequent pregnancy if there is a history of infertility. If the woman is pregnant for a second time since you have been trying to conceive, this may seem particularly unfair. Friends' or relatives' pregnancies that correspond to your own pregnancy loss are especially hard to bear.

During a friend's pregnancy, there are special challenges for both of you, requiring honesty and tact. Some friendships are secure enough to withstand a temporary hiatus if the reason is understood and the relationship valued enough:

> Although most people continue to say all of the wrong things, there have been others who have been wonderful. My closest friend was able to understand enough to forgive me for ignoring her during most of her second pregnancy.

One woman who was able to transcend her emotional ambivalence toward a friend's pregnancy received a remarkable testimony of her goodwill:

> She has recently told me that she and her husband have discussed the possibility of having another baby and giving it to us. No words could describe the love that I felt, although I did explain to her that we were nowhere near the point of medically giving up and that it was a incredible selfless thought but the idea is emotionally and legally unrealistic.

Being unable to wholeheartedly share in a friend's joy may cause you to have doubts about yourself. Some women deplore that they cannot rise above their own situation to celebrate a friend's good fortune. Although this is a normal, temporary protective response to infertility, some women chastise themselves for having become selfish and uncaring. They have not become jealous or envious individuals; their feelings pertain only to others' fertility. Their ambivalence is perhaps best captured in the phrase "I'm happy for you, but sad for myself."

When the pregnancy is within the family, some of you may find that your joy predominates, while for others this is the hardest scenario. Feelings about your siblings and even birth order can come into play at this time; it can be particularly hard to see a younger sibling going ahead in building his or her family. If you have a single child, you may be thrilled that your child will have cousins close in age. Infertility, however, can also rekindle long-dormant sibling rivalry.[4] You might feel jealous if your child is no longer the youngest grandchild, feeling that he or she has been displaced by a fertile sibling's child. If your sister or brother claims a crib that has been in the family, asks for your unused baby items, or chooses a name for the child that you had fantasied about using, feelings can be especially strained. Serving as a godparent to your nieces or nephews may be a bittersweet honor.

Attending Family Events and Baby Showers

An ongoing quandary is what role to play at family and social gatherings that revolve around children and pregnancy. The desire to have your child participate may be strong, even though the get-togethers may be painful for you. You don't want to lose out on being with your family; however, at times it is difficult to take part. To what degree the family understands and is sensitive to your needs may determine how you handle these situations. While childless couples might more readily opt out of such occasions, as parents, particularly of single children, most likely you want your child to spend time with relatives whenever possible. Focusing on your child's enjoyment of the event can help to counter your own more mixed feelings.

Another common dilemma is whether or not to attend baby showers for pregnant relatives, friends, or co-workers. There is no reason you must attend an event that will be painful for you. All that should be necessary is an acknowledgment that while you would like to attend, you're afraid it isn't possible. Unfortunately, in many families such a response would not be accepted. Just as a rational person would not repeatedly put a hand over a hot burner, so too is there no need to inflict emotional pain on yourself. It is difficult to claim the right to be self-sustaining, often feeling that you owe it to the pregnant woman to celebrate with her. But as the saying goes, "I don't want to rain on your parade, but I don't have to march in it either."

While you are experiencing infertility, it is natural to feel vulnerable and self-protective. This does not mean that you have ceased to be loving aunts or uncles, or that you have become self-centered and uncaring. You are simply respecting your temporary limitations and later will be able to resume normal family roles. It is important that you feel comfortable about avoiding painful encounters and not take such normal feelings as further evidence of failure. Often one partner will feel that there are social obligations that his or her spouse should fulfill. Although you may have an intuitive sense of what you can or cannot handle, sometimes it is useful to have official sanction to do what is in your own best interest.

Aline Zoldbrod, author of *Men, Women, and Infertility: Intervention and Treatment Strategies*, describes how therapists can give you "very scientific-sounding permission to avoid the problem situation." Simply stated, certain stimuli, such as baby showers or first-birthday parties, can be expected to result in negative outcomes, such as jealousy or depression. Given this knowledge, the best way to avoid the unwanted outcome is to control (or avoid) the stimulus.[5] In other words, avoid events you anticipate will be uncomfortable, and explain to family and spouse why you are doing so.

Being self-protective can have many benefits and in some situations is clearly the wisest course, at least for the time being:

> One thing which really helped me was the decision that I really could stay home from situations or groups that were too painful for me to take part in. I withdrew from one group when the majority of women kept complaining how awful it was to be pregnant, after I had just shared our struggle with infertility. For several years, I did not go to baby showers. I just knew that it was too hard emotionally and better for me to stay away while others rejoiced.

Such a decision, while not easy to reach, can be liberating, self-sustaining, and one way in which you can regain some control over your life:

> Take care of yourself, first. You can't worry about hurting other people by not going to baby showers, namings, etc. Your mental health comes first. If other people can't/don't understand why it's too difficult for you to be around them, it's their problem, not yours.

On the other hand, some women feel that attending such events is a way to prove themselves and that by not going, they will be admitting defeat and withdrawing from the club of fertile women. Others go to please their spouses, particularly if an in-law is pregnant. If for whatever reason you would feel worse by not going or if the cost in self-esteem or disapproval from others is too great, attending may be the best choice; ideally, however, you should try to decide on the basis of what is best for you, not the person being honored.

Before attending what is anticipated to be a difficult occasion, it is helpful to visualize what the experience will be like. You might picture yourself there and think about how you might respond to various questions or comments. You could line up the support of another family member or friend to serve as a buffer or just to have someone there who realizes what you are going through. It is helpful to remind yourself that you may leave at any time; putting in a brief appearance is certainly an option. Preparing ahead of time emotionally for such an event may be time well spent; some women report that many of the anticipated problems never materialized and that they felt more confident about responding to the ones that did.

Coping with Insensitive Remarks

The RESOLVE newsletter once ran a column along the lines of "Snappy Comebacks to Stupid Comments." Similarly, an inevitable topic for discussion in support groups is the painful remarks made by others. One of the best arguments for making the effort to educate others is the hope that knowledge will cut down on the types of uninformed responses reported below.

Infertility elicits a range of sexual advice and jokes. Following a miscarriage, one woman received a card from a female cousin with Mickey Mouse on front saying, "Have fun trying again." A woman describes typical remarks from those who just don't get it: "People would make comments about how lucky we were not to have to use birth control, that we should relax, or how much fun we should have in the process."

Ironically, religious beliefs can be the source of some hurt feelings. One woman was told by someone pregnant with her fourth child who knew of her infertility that "God knew who should have children." Others have been told that infertility is "God's way of testing [them]." Another woman reasoned that "it is not nature's (or God's) preoccupation" who can or can't or should have babies; however, her friends continued to attribute the infertility to God's will. She puts the matter in another perspective:

> It is so easy for friends, with their wished-for two or three children safely in hand, to voice their opinion that "if God wanted you to have another

baby, you would." Well, if God didn't want us to discover the miracle of assisted reproduction, we wouldn't have. If God didn't want humans to use surrogacy as a means to have children, He wouldn't have created the caring women who are willing to make this contribution.

The desire to blame the victim (e.g., "If only you relaxed," "It's God's will") may be people's attempt to rationalize why such a problem cannot happen to them. It is less frightening to others to feel there is a reason for the infertility than to believe it is a random occurrence that could affect them as well.

The lack of respect for the privacy of those undergoing infertility treatment also reflects insensitivity. Some people ask too many personal questions and/or ask about matters that should remain private. Others treat the subject so matter-of-factly that they cause embarrassment, such as the librarian who loudly commented on the theme of the infertility books being checked out.

Some women recall either being referred to as a "jinx" or being treated as such and avoided by pregnant friends and associates as though the infertility were contagious. Certainly, infertile women can be a reminder that things do go wrong.

The lack of understanding is widespread, encompassing not only relatives and friends but also the clergy and even some doctors. One priest tried to comfort a woman by likening her situation to that of a nun; she did not find the comparison useful:

> Even the priest I went to was next to useless. He told me, "There are more ways to glorify God than having children—just look at me and the other religious, such as nuns"! As if he didn't *choose* his life. I did *not choose* to never have another child.

Even doctors may fail to realize how emotionally charged the condition is: An endocrinologist announced with no sense of irony that he had "good news," meaning that the body was working fine, adding that there was nothing he could do to increase the fertility.

Communicating with Family and Friends

Setting limits on attending baby showers or on subjecting yourself to insensitive remarks is a way to preserve relationships. But establishing limits requires revealing not only your infertility but also your emotional needs. While you may reason that it is best to keep quiet in the interests of family harmony, often this is not the result. As Barbara Eck Menning astutely observes, "Remarks, often very direct and personal, are usually endured until a point of pain is reached where the couple react angrily, or withdraw in silence with their secret of infertility."[6] She goes on to explain that when people keep their infertility secret or keep quiet, fearing that others won't understand, they are setting themselves up for "one painful encounter after another" or else isolation in an attempt to feel "safe." Instead, she recommends that you tell people about the infertility so that they will have no excuse for making insensitive comments. She advises couples to point out to others instances in which their remarks are inappropriate or hurtful and to refuse to answer intrusive questions.

Even occasional angry outbursts in response to thoughtless remarks by those close to you can be worked through. In fact, confronting those who have been thoughtless can be positive. A book on dealing with pregnancy loss states this case; the wider applicability is apparent:

> You may derive a sense of accomplishment by confronting people whose responses are inconsiderate, when you feel up to it. Thoughtless comments or silences present an opportunity to educate others about pregnancy loss and how it should be handled in our society.

It quotes one woman who explains:

> I felt so passionately about telling people how important it was to make a connection to us in our grief, . . . it became almost a crusade for me.[7]

While it may seem unfair that those with the problem must educate others as to how to be sensitive, Menning feels that this is often the case: "A person with a problem—any problem—unfortunately has the burden of explaining to others the nature of the problem, and how others may be helpful." She offers a narrative example to illustrate:

> I approached an intersection where a blind boy of about eighteen was attempting to cross a busy street. I came to his side and . . . said, "Would you like me to help you across the street?" He answered with such confidence that I was taken aback. He said, "Yes, if you will just take a firm grip on my elbow here and tell me when we reach the op-

posite curb, I would be very appreciative." After I left him at the other side I thought for a long while about this encounter. I realized that he had helped *me* to help him, in a way that made us both feel good. I think this is the same with infertility, but more difficult, as our problem is invisible. We have to help others to help us.[8]

There are ways to "help others to help." You can bring up the infertility if you feel like talking about it; in this way, you let it be known that it is something that you can discuss. Just as you can initiate discussions, so too you can decide whether or not, where, and when to deal with the issue. Some settings are just not appropriate, and there are times when you can't risk being vulnerable. Groundrules are helpful to all parties in negotiating what is acceptable and appreciated (e.g., "We'll tell you if there is any news").

Relatives and friends often feel frustrated about how best to respond, feeling that they are in a no-win situation: When they ask questions, they are seen as prying, or they don't ask and are thought to be indifferent. Some people avoid the topic out of feelings of helplessness or the lack of knowledge of the right thing to say. Many feel that they must respond to a problem with a solution; they don't realize that you need to vent your feelings and have them acknowledged and accepted; you do not expect others to cheer you up, and it is usually a mistake to try.

You can try to legitimize the reactions of those around you. Family members may suppress their own disappointment, feeling that it is disloyal to the grandchild they have or that they will make you feel worse. Acknowledge that you realize it is hard to know what to say, let it be known that you don't need "magical solutions," and tell them what would be helpful. Knowing you don't expect solutions or cheering up may enable others to listen more empathically, without worrying about saying the wrong thing.

Many of the common trivializing remarks grow out of the tendency to try to show that things aren't as bad as they seem or could be worse. One woman captures the mismatch between people's responses and what she needed to hear:

> I really didn't expect people to become emotionally involved, but just to give me an *acknowledgment* of the pain I was feeling. I felt that time and time again, my feelings were considered invalid, something to be

brushed aside. Another common reaction was trying to cheer me up so that I would feel better. . . . Hardly anyone said to me, "Yes, it *is* awful," or "I can see this is really hard for you," or . . . simply "I'm sorry this happened to you." It has taken a great deal of communication on my part to let people know what to say and do. . . . Attempting to make light of the situation denies the reality, . . . as well as my right to grieve.

If I had to choose one thing to change in those having to cope with someone going through secondary infertility, it would be to simply acknowledge their feelings, no matter what they are. It is devastating to feel like you're alone with your emotions, that somehow they are wrong or weird or even crazy. . . . Naturally, no one will feel the pain as deeply as I do—I wouldn't expect them to.

Another woman elaborates that she would like others to know

how hurtful their statements can be when they try to magically solve your problems by saying things like "You just need to relax and it will happen," "You just need a vacation," or "When you stop thinking about it, that's when it will happen." All the "I had a friend" stories can be just as hurtful. It seems that everyone has a friend that got pregnant "just when she. . . ." Statements such as these are all well meaning, but a person going through this does not need to hear these things; they need a supportive friend, one who will listen and not try to provide magical solutions.

Understanding not only the medical realities of infertility but also the common emotional reactions provides others with a perspective on your experience. Witnessing the anger and depression that often temporarily accompanies infertility can be frightening if it is not seen as part of your healing process. Witnessing your pain can cause relatives and friends to feel overwhelmed and helpless. The knowledge that you have other supports and resources available can be reassuring to them.

Last, know when to cut your losses. As Barbara Eck Menning puts it, "There are some people who, like racists and sexists, are hopeless cases for education. These people are probably best avoided."[9] Such people can't always be avoided, particularly if they are relatives or co-workers; however, if and when they do make hurtful remarks, it may help to consider the source and try to ignore the remarks as reflecting negatively on the speaker rather than on you. On the other hand, don't be too quick to write someone off as unsalvageable; with the proper feedback, even someone who previously had no clue about infertility may suddenly "get it."

RESOLVE, Inc., has an excellent fact sheet that provides those concerned about someone coping with infertility with suggestions on ways to help. Giving a family member or friend this handout with a note saying "Because I know you care and want to help" is a positive way to broach the subject without reproaching the person for prior insensitivity. Newspaper articles can highlight the issue in a more general way, while hopefully laying the groundwork for discussion and eventual understanding.

Describing an ideal way of communicating needs, the RESOLVE fact sheet advises family and friends to

> ask them how you can be supportive. Do they want you to ask how things are going or do they want you to wait until they initiate discussion? Would they like you to accompany them to the clinic? Would it be helpful for you to bring over the evening meal, particularly after certain procedures or surgeries? If they don't know, encourage them to think about what they expect so that they can let you know. This acknowledges to the couple that they are the authority on what they need, when they need it and from whom they would like to receive it.[10]

Hopefully, you will be able to find the support you need and deserve from those close to you. Still, it is crucial that if your usual sources of support are unable to respond, you find alternative resources, whether from professionals or peer support groups. One couple who felt let down by those close to them described their solution:

> We ended up seeing a psychologist who had experienced infertility, and that was helpful. It just felt so good to have someone give credence to our pain and to listen to us. It did bother me that we had to pay someone to do what we felt our family and friends should have been able to do.

They were, however, able to find support and may find that they can forgive and reconnect with family and friends once this crisis is resolved.

5

Caught between Two Worlds

Having one foot in the fertile world and one foot in the infertile world is like being nowhere
—Woman describing the isolation of secondary infertility

This statement eloquently captures the crux of the secondary infertility dilemma. Parents experiencing secondary infertility are uniquely isolated. Although you are infertile, you are not childless; although you are parents, you are not currently fertile. The feeling is that "people with primary infertility do not want to hear from those with a child. Normally fertile people can't understand what the fuss is about." One woman with recurring infertility considers the experience much worse this time, because she feels alienated from other women:

> I feel much more isolated from other women now. I don't belong with women who don't have kids and don't want them; we simply can't relate. I don't belong with women who want children but can't get pregnant; I actually have what they want most—how could I not feel satisfied? I don't ever feel like a full-fledged member of the Mommy Club; I only have one—what could I possibly know of unplanned pregnancy, sibling rivalry, divided loyalty, or even fatigue?

There is no natural support network for those of you with secondary infertility. It is difficult for both childless friends and other parents to empathize with your feelings of pain and loss. Somehow you must fulfill your role as parents while shielding yourselves from constant reminders of lost fertility.

A Hidden Loss

Many couples delay seeking treatment or support for this problem by rationalizing that they obviously are not infertile; after all, they live with a daily proof of their fertility.

> I remember the first time I saw *Infertility* marked as my diagnosis; . . . certainly, it did not truly apply to me. But as each failed cycle went by, I was forced to realize that yes, I was infertile. A strange condition to accept when I saw my own flesh-and-blood child. I had given birth to her, I had been pregnant, and yet the reality of being able to do that now seemed beyond me.

Secondary infertility appears to be a contradiction in terms. If it were a real problem, why haven't you read or heard about it? One woman searched for information:

> I went to the library to try to educate myself on what was happening and hopefully find a little comfort and direction. I was frustrated because infertility books seemed to confront only primary infertility. I found very little information about secondary infertility, and then it was mainly newspaper or magazine articles. . . . I had for a very long time the mislead[ing] idea that my infertile friends with no children were really in for a hard time because I had become pregnant before and obviously would again.

You may feel that you are fair game to those inquiring, innocently or not, about your family planning intentions. While there is some recognition that couples may not be childless by choice, there is no such understanding toward those who have "proven" fertility. Unknowing, others pry and make assumptions that are unfounded and hurtful, such as the following laments:

> The callousness of that question—"When are you are going to have another one?"—[and] the invasion of privacy it entails were very offensive to me. The assumption that I wanted "only one" for selfish reasons also upset me. I particularly resented [it] when adults asked my daughter . . . these questions.

Ironically, today many couples choose to limit their family size for reasons that are valid and acceptable to them. If you hide your secondary infertility, you may have to defend yourself against stereo-types that in no way apply. The last thing you want or need is someone trying to sell you on having more children or accusing you of selfishness for not doing so.

> I don't like people thinking that I only wanted one child, because (a) I wanted to focus on my career, (b) I wanted to keep the house clean eas-ily, (c) I'm not that crazy about children but my husband deserved at least one. The reasons most people have given to me that they chose to just have one seem selfish, and I don't like people assuming I'm like that because I had one child and could "obviously" have more but didn't. Few people understand secondary infertility until they experience it.

The reluctance to share the problem with others is not, however, the only reason that the loss remains hidden and unsupported. Un-fortunately, some couples reveal their pain only to find that others minimize their loss due to a lack of knowledge and understanding of the problem.

Lack of Validation

Even when you share news of the infertility with others, you may still receive little or no validation of this loss. In fact, many reac-tions blame the victim for wanting another child by admonishing you to be grateful for the child you have. Such insensitivity can be maddening:

> Practically nothing would enrage me more than hearing . . . "At least you already have a child." . . . No one would say to a child who has lost one parent, "Well, at least you have one parent."

Another woman responds to some dismissive comments she received:

> I *know* I'm blessed. People seem to get mad at me for not feeling grate-ful for the child I have. "You are lucky you have Claire," they say. . . . Everyone has a story about a *worse* situation—"Thank God you have Claire," "Be thankful you are not dying," "Some people can never have one," "Many choose to have only one," "It's easier to have one."

One woman describes how her diverse roles serve both to obscure the loss and to cause others to minimize it:

Since I work full-time outside my home and recently turned forty, many co-workers may assume that my husband and I have completed our family. When I discuss my secondary infertility, . . . some compare my infertility with that of a [childless] co-worker's wife and have said, . . . "It would be worse if you didn't have any kids." At some level, I agree with them that it may be different, but . . . I feel like this potential loss deserves empathy and concern.

Feeling Guilty

Feeling guilty about mourning your loss is one common pitfall for all secondarily infertile couples. The following account touches on many of the emotions:

I longed to know a child was again growing inside of me, to feel it move, to hold it close and nurse again. There were people who would say, "You have one child; why can't you just be content?" I would look at David, think about what a miracle he was, and chastise myself for wanting more rather than being thankful. While reading books on infertility, I would think, You at least have one; they have none. But that never took away my desire for another child. I needed to talk to someone . . . experiencing secondary infertility. A number of friends had lived through [primary] infertility, and . . . they didn't know exactly what I was feeling. Sometimes I even felt guilty being with them, because I had a child and they still had been unable to bear one.

The guilt may be exacerbated for those with recurring infertility who may have bargained that just one child would make them happy. One woman relates her mixed emotions:

Finally, after three-and-a-half years and seven cycles of Clomid, we were pregnant. . . . She was our miracle baby. I always said that if I just had one baby I'd be happy.

Now it is three-and-a-half years later. Sara is no longer a baby and will be attending preschool. . . . I also feel very guilty for wanting another child because I do have one, and I consider her my little miracle. Maybe it's selfish to ask for another miracle. . . . [My husband] feels I'm not always thankful for what I have—but "normal" people who have two or three kids aren't thankful for the blessing they have either.

Although it is sometimes referred to as one-child infertility, secondary infertility occurs after any number of children. Couples with more than one child are particularly prone to feel guilty or selfish, although they too have not been able to achieve their desired family size. A mother of two characterizes her position:

Heaped onto all this mess was the guilt I felt because I had already had two children—one of each sex. What if I had none kept tormenting me. I didn't feel I had the right to want more when so many people had no children. Many people with two-child families could not understand my desire for another. It is very difficult for people to understand who are happy in their two-child families why you can't be happy in yours. If there is little sympathy for the secondary infertility couple who have one child, then there is no sympathy for the secondary infertility couple who have two children.

Another woman who lost her first child and then had two more children candidly discusses her ambivalence about having another child, her feelings about being unable to complete her family, and how her position is perceived by others:

First, with secondary infertility, there is an ambivalence about having more children. This is an internal ambivalence that I think any parent understands. Some days, you wonder if you even want the ones you already have! Other times, they are so wonderful that you want to clone them. For me too, I see such differences in my two living children that I really want to see what another one will be like.

This internal ambivalence is harder because of the lack of social support for having more children. In the infertile community, I feel like I'm being greedy to want three children. When you're around people who are trying so desperately to become parents at all, you can't give voice to the range of feelings you are experiencing. We have attended very few RESOLVE meetings, feeling that we would be out of place. From the fertile world, we get the messages of how lucky we are and how we should be happy with what we have. Especially now that we have a child of each gender, most people assume that we have the "ideal family." Since we lost our first child, we will never have our own personal ideal family, but now I feel like I'm missing the beginning and the end of my family.

Assuming you were fertile, you may have made what you then considered to be prudent decisions about family planning and now regret not having had children closer together while everything was "working." If you terminated a pregnancy, this can occasion special feelings of guilt and even cause some people to question whether their infertility is a punishment. Consider the circumstances of the woman whose experience is related below, who has been trying for seven years to have another child.

> It was a life-threatening delivery. . . . I had over one hundred stitches, . . . blood transfusions, . . . [and] was in the hospital for nearly two weeks. Five months later, when I still could not sit comfortably for any length of time, I unbelievably became pregnant. The thought threw me into such a panic: I couldn't imagine going through birth so soon. Without much thought except the fear of repeating a horrid experience before I'd had time to heal, I had an abortion.
>
> By the time my boy was a year and a half, loving him like crazy, wanting to achieve my husband's and my original wish for a large family and particularly seeking out a new doctor who would assure me that if I carried another disproportionately large baby, he would perform a C-section, I started trying for another baby. I'm still trying. . . .
>
> There are so few people on this earth that know I've had an abortion. This subject has obviously been a source of awful pain, and I spent many hours at the counselor's office trying to keep the act in perspective and not hate myself for that decision.

Other couples conceive a subsequent pregnancy easily, only to receive news through amniocentesis or ultrasound of a genetic defect. Some decide to terminate the pregnancy, feeling this is in the best interests of their family and hoping that another pregnancy that is not affected will soon ensue. Unfortunately, this is not always the case.

You may know intellectually that you did not cause your infertility; however, the feeling of having been judged and singled out for punishment can linger irrationally and compound your pain. Clearly, though, infertility is random and not a punishment, just as fertility is not a reward.

Special Situations

Some people may be both secondarily infertile and currently childless. This population includes men or women who may have had a child in a former marriage and do not have custody. Often the fertile partner in these couples feels guilt that he or she was able to have a child in a former relationship, but not in the current partnership in which he or she is emotionally invested. Another hidden group is women who make an adoption plan for their child and later find themselves infertile. Having given birth and being without a child, they do not fit easily into any category. For instance:

> Ten years ago, I conceived out of wedlock. My son was adopted through a Catholic adoption agency. Now married for five years, my husband and I have struggled with the sometimes overwhelming feeling of "why then, but not now?" I know, for me, the added burden of my secret past and child has at times caused almost unbearable pain.

Yet another group that is not immune from secondary infertility is bereaved parents. While this is a painful possibility for any parent to contemplate, it can and does occur, as the following account attests:

> My ambivalence [about having children] disappeared once Stephen was born. Although he was a colicky, intense baby, I fell in love with him. Having children became a lot more appealing to me once I had one. Stephen became ill with a cold when he was two-and-a-half months old and died from complications. Although we knew we didn't want to have another child until we had begun to recover from his death, the very day he died we said that it would be a worse tragedy if he were the only baby we were ever able to have. I suppose this scenario is somewhat unusual, but I know several bereaved parents who have also experienced infertility, and it is a combination of hurt that I wouldn't wish on my worst enemies!

While all parents worry about the well-being of their children, perhaps particularly if that child is an only child, as is discussed in Chapter 7, some parents have a firstborn who is medically at risk such as this mother who is experiencing secondary infertility:

> My daughter . . . was not expected to live past two weeks; she came home after spending three months in the hospital. Her prognosis was not good. . . . Today we are not out of the woods, but Marie is a beautiful, active four-and-a-half-year-old. She has 20 percent kidney function and will eventually need a transplant. . . . After Marie was born, I was very ambivalent about having another baby. Part of me was terrified to go through it all again; a part of me was scared Marie would die

and I'd have nothing. . . . My fears that Marie will one day get sicker and may die are not unfounded in reality.

Dealing with Isolation

Parents experiencing infertility are uniquely isolated: belonging to the world of neither the fertile nor the childless. You do not fit easily in any niche. You may feel that you have nowhere to find others like you. You may find yourself searching for peers:

> I'm constantly looking for one-child families (I even wrote to Hillary Clinton!), and I don't find many among my friends. . . . Just yesterday, I met a woman with a little girl Abby's age, at the beach. I found myself thinking, Great, another only child—but just then, her older son came running over.

Many parents of one child report casting around for others in the same situation: studying school directories, eyeballing crowds for families that look like them, etc. Through RESOLVE, playgroups have been formed of mothers experiencing secondary infertility and their children. Some RESOLVE chapters run support groups specifically for those experiencing secondary infertility; others have a person-to-person contact system. (The role of RESOLVE is discussed more fully in Chapter 10.) This provides a valuable resource to many, as the following testifys:

> I was going through a very terrible time and it lasted for about three years. I joined RESOLVE, and limited my emotional "letting down my fences" to other infertile people who understood. The "fertile" world was too hard to deal with.

> I called the RESOLVE hotline . . . and spoke with another woman (she is still my friend) with secondary infertility. She encouraged me to join a weekly support group, which was mostly comprised of primary infertility. The group was supportive and caring (despite the fact that I already had a child), and in many way I credit that experience with getting me past infertility.

On the other hand, one RESOLVE member cautions:

> One drawback [of joining RESOLVE], however, is that people get pregnant whom you've relied on for support, and then you feel isolated

all over again. . . . This is so painful for me to deal with. . . . It's better not to get *too* involved with people, because there's always the chance they'll get pregnant and you're the "odd one out."

Further, if you have devoted yourself to parenting at the expense of your career, you may be particularly isolated. Some parents, usually mothers, may have forgone career advancement, taken part-time work, or taken time-out to parent, thereby cutting off other potential sources of personal gratification and support. If you work outside the home, however, you may have found that the office, rather than being a respite from the world of the fertile, also appears to be populated by pregnant women or mothers who talk about their babies.

Impact of the Fertile Community

Many, if not most, childless infertile couples isolate themselves from those with children. They may find that they have more in common with single friends from work than with peers who have become child-oriented. Yet, when you are experiencing secondary infertility, you are yourselves child-oriented and have left the world of child-free activities behind. Often you live in neighborhoods conducive to young families and in many ways have organized your lives and social networks around children.

Ironically, those who may have been the greatest support to you in parenting your first child may now become the greatest source of hurt as they go on to repeat your previously shared parenting experience with subsequent children. Lacking any infertility background themselves, they may be at a loss as to how to comfort you and may unwittingly and without malice compound the pain. One woman reports such a well-meant attempt which backfired:

> It felt like Alice attempted to "solve" my infertility crisis by bringing me [her] baby for a few days. She had *no* idea how it felt for me to be in this baby's presence. I think she thought "sharing" her baby with me would somehow help. It only hurt. It was horribly painful trying to uphold my hostess role while also feeling so desperately jealous and angry. . . . A fresh-faced thirdborn—my namesake yet—thrust before my envious face.

The feeling of having been left behind is exacerbated when peers go on to have not only second children but third or more children. One woman describes the emphasis on fertility in her community:

> I live in a religious community where three to four children are the average. I am the only one here with one child past the age of one-and-a-half. The thought of dealing with people makes me paralyzed. I want to climb in my bed and never get out. . . . And the community I live in is small. Everyone knows everything. All the women ever talk about is who's pregnant, did Rachel have the baby yet, and then birth stories are compared over and over. I'm tired of smiling quietly through it all and pretending it doesn't matter. I'm tired of going to celebrations and putting on a happy face. . . .
>
> It seems that everyone I know is pregnant. All my friends who got married when I did or even after me have two or more children. One's pregnant with number three; two are pregnant with their fourth.

You cannot easily follow the conventional advice to limit painful encounters with pregnant women and newborns. Picking up your child at nursery school may feel like running an emotional gantlet. Participating in a parent-toddler class may not be a fun-filled activity, but rather an act of courage. One woman summarizes the dilemma:

> All the infertility books say to stay away from children if you can't handle it, but I'm forced into the fertile world—pregnant neighbors, friends, etc. Also, everyone assumes that since you have one child, having a second should be a snap. I wish I had a dime for the times each person has asked about the next baby. I've gotten pretty good at being evasive.

Status in the Infertile Community

A recent survey of RESOLVE members documents that only a small percentage (3 to 5 percent) of its members are dealing with secondary infertility. Given the high incidence of secondary infertility (the majority of the infertile), this disparity is striking. This low level of affiliation may reflect a lack of awareness of services, as well as a reluctance to identify with infertility. Some individuals who accept the unwelcome idea of being secondarily infertile wonder if they will be accepted as such. While RESOLVE, Inc. recognizes the needs of this population and wishes to serve them, the fact that such a small number of those with secondary infertility join the organization makes it difficult to provide services specifically for them and parents often attend programs with predominantly childless members. The following accounts illustrate the potentially trying dynamics:

> I went to the local RESOLVE group for nearly a year before I let it slip out that I had a child already. The women there felt like they had more grief because they had no child, and it was hard to try to compare who felt worse.

> Even though RESOLVE was my sanity-saver, I still experienced "discrimination" whenever a member would discover I was already a mother. It was as if they could not understand how I could feel the pangs of infertility when I already had a child. So I limited my mention of my son around certain people. It was like "What right do you have to claim infertility has devastated your life?"

Being isolated within a support group is a cruel irony and may feel like the ultimate rejection. While some RESOLVE chapters and medical clinics are able to run separate support groups for those with children, often this is not feasible. Even when offered, such groups sometimes take a long time to fill and require members to travel long distances. Combining women or couples with primary and secondary infertility can be difficult for both group leaders and participants. It is necessary to transcend differences and recognize the shared feelings of loss in order to be able to relate empathetically to one another. Openness about having a child is necessary to establish trust; however, such a revelation is hard to make. A RESOLVE fact sheet discusses this dilemma:

> I was very excited about this group, because at last I was going to meet other women who were infertile. I never gave it a thought that my infertility was different from theirs until after the first session. . . . I felt so close to the members of the group that I was afraid their knowledge of our child would separate me from them. So I hid it from them and never mentioned it. . . . I knew they must know the truth, that it wasn't fair to hide it from them. I so badly wanted and needed to be part of the group that I couldn't risk losing their support and understanding by

telling them the truth. I had gone almost three years without this much-needed support, and I felt now I was going to lose it.

I could feel some anger and hostility from others in the group; they did not understand how I could be infertile. Fortunately, through several sessions, we were able to work things out and I was accepted into the group.[1]

Issues Unique to Secondary Infertility

This section does not attempt to weigh or rate the pain of primary vs. secondary infertility. Both are painful, and the pain varies in each individual situation. The following account ruefully describes the irony of a couple having taken their fertility for granted:

> We assumed that because everything had gone rather smoothly with this pregnancy, a future one would go the same way. We decided that we wanted two children about three years apart. . . . We were so sure that everything would go as smoothly as the first time that we even decided what month we wanted the baby to be born. When we didn't get pregnant in the first several months, we elected to use protection for a couple of months so we wouldn't have a baby born near Christmas. With four years of infertility under my belt [now], I can hardly believe that we thought we had so much control that we could determine when our next child would be born!

Couples with recurring infertility are in a position to describe what each form of infertility has meant in their own lives. In the following account, the writer, who has had a recurring fertility problem, reports that on the whole, the secondary infertility experience has been easier for her; however, she describes some "special challenges":

> Since I also suffered from primary infertility, . . . even during my daughter's infancy, I was aware that this might be the only baby that I would ever have. I certainly hoped that I would be able to conceive again, but I knew that the chances were that I would have to go through some effort to do so.
>
> I began treatment when my daughter was three-and-a-half, and for me this time has been, on the whole, much easier. Although my husband, my daughter, and I all want a baby very much, there have not been the desperation and fear of never being able to be a mother. There

have been many tears and some terrible disappointments, but always I know that we are already a family and that we could be OK as a one-child family.

Although, in general, dealing with trying to get pregnant this time has been easier, there have been some special challenges. . . . When we did not have a child, there was no question of what the priority was, but now we must balance the needs of the child we have against our hope of having another. In addition to the special complications of dealing with infertility treatment when one already has a child, I have felt somewhat less support this time around. . . .

As a woman who has dealt with both primary and secondary infertility, I have always known that I was very fortunate to be able to have even one child. . . . If our current attempt is not successful, we will be faced with coming to terms with not having another child. If that happens, I will grieve, but my grief will always be tempered by thankfulness for the tremendous blessing of my daughter.

In general, as parents experiencing infertility, whether or not you have a prior history of infertility, you inevitably perceive the loss through your viewpoint as parents. The following analogy illustrates this perspective:

When you don't have any children, there is certainly a loss. But when I compare my yearning for a second and third child to what I wished when I was pregnant with my first, there is no comparison, because before you have a child, you really don't know what to expect. It's like wanting to go to France and you've never been there. You've heard it's great, and you hope it's great, but you don't really know what it'll be like. Well, I've been "there" and now I'm terrified I won't be able to go back. I know that my little boy has filled parts of my heart I didn't dream were lacking, and I'd like what everyone else seems to have so effortlessly—a family size my husband and I are in control of.

In a similar vein:

I know it is extremely painful for the totally childless couple, but in a way, it's almost easier. Because for people with secondary infertility, they were actually given the experience of what it feels like to be pregnant, to go through labor, and to see their child being born. But then for some unknown reason it was taken away forever.

Miscarriages may also be experienced differently by different people, depending on their fertility and parenting history. For some fertile women, a pregnancy loss is exactly that: a lost pregnancy which they assume will be readily repeated. The pregnancy itself may have been a cause for excitement, and much attention may have been paid to bodily changes and the anticipated delivery. But for other women, among them mothers and infertile women, a pregnancy loss feels like the death of a longed-for child. Once you have had a child, a subsequent pregnancy is more likely to be visualized in terms of an actual child. One mother wrote a letter to memorialize what she considered to be her child, lost at eleven weeks' gestation:

> I wondered if you'd be like Sara when she was born. I couldn't wait to nurse you, to hold your floppy head. . . . I started putting away Sara's toys for you and looking over her clothes to see what you could wear. . . . I was going to take you everywhere with me in the Snugli—to the beach, to school with Sara. You would have loved having Sara for a sister. . . .
>
> It's a very personal, private loss. So many people never even knew you existed. It's very lonely mourning by ourselves.
>
> People say I'm lucky to have your sister (and I know I am) and that I'll have other pregnancies (maybe I will). But what about *you*? No one can ever take the place of what you might have been.

Another woman had such a fully realized image of her embryos as her potential children that she wrote a letter "To My Unborn Children" after her embryos were transferred into her uterus:

> When I look at your brother[s] . . . , I dream about how wonderful it would be to sit back and enjoy you the same way I dearly love them. I marvel at their uniqueness, and . . . I pray that you get the chance to see birth and development as they have.
>
> I still mourn your two siblings who never made it to the seven-week sonogram. And I also wonder about the three embryos who didn't make it. But whether one or all five of you make it through all the hurdles down the road, you will still be my children and I love you all the same.

It is clear that to this woman, as to many mothers, an unsuccessful treatment cycle represents not just a failed medical procedure but also a tangible loss of a longed-for child. A mother who has suffered five miscarriages differentiates her feelings from the conventional medical perspective:

> I have considered each of my pregnancies to be a baby, a tiny, living human being that I love very much. I realize that, from a medical standpoint, it isn't a baby yet. But as soon as I see a positive pregnancy test, I think, I'm going to have a *baby*,—not an ovum, fetus, or anything else. This belief has led to disagreements between some of my doctors, nurses, certain friends, and family members. It is very difficult for some people to understand how I could grieve over "something I never saw, held, felt kick, etc." I do because each baby was a member of our family, even if for a very brief time. . . . When each baby died, I felt unbelievable pain and sorrow, as well as a deep feeling of loss.

Addressing the relative pain of primary and secondary infertility, a RESOLVE support group leader and clinical social worker, Judith Calica, writing in the *Chicago Parent*, said it best: "The pain is real and no less legitimate than anyone else's. Since none of us lives comparative lives, only our own lives, our pain is our pain and it really does hurt."[2] It is a question not of establishing a hierarchy of suffering, but rather of acknowledging to yourselves and others the real pain that exists and trying to find ways to cope with your unique infertility status and your singular position of having "one foot in each world."

II

Parenting During Secondary Infertility

6

Helping Your Child Cope with Secondary Infertility

I am far from accepting the unfairness of the infertility as it relates to my son.

—Mother concerned about the impact of secondary infertility on her child

One of the hardest parts of experiencing infertility as a parent is the worry about its effect on your existing child or children. Just as infertility regardless of diagnosis is considered a "couple problem," so too must secondary infertility to some extent be thought of as a family crisis. It is difficult to cope with not only your own and your spouse's reactions but also your child's. The following explores the implications of infertility as a three-way proposition:

> This is another aspect of secondary infertility that makes it in some ways more complex than primary infertility. In primary infertility, you really have only yourselves (you and your husband) to think about, although obviously other family and friends are affected. But with secondary, in addition to your own grief, you have major concerns about the child you have and the impact on her of not having a sibling. This creates another level of stress and guilt in not being able to give her everything you would like to.

A woman with a recurring infertility finds decision making harder the second time around, questioning how much money, time, and effort should be invested; how many chances she and her husband should take with surgery; and, above all, "Is any of this fair to the child we have? Does he feel the stress in the house, and does he understand why? . . . My son is one more person who is hurt by my failure."

Why Your Children Need to Be Told

You may believe that your child's life is *not* affected by the infertility. This may be true, depending on your child's age and how you have been affected; some parents, however, prefer to believe this is the case rather than face the problem it presents. It is very hard to objectively assess the impact of your pain on your child. Most parents hope to provide their children with a trouble-free childhood and feel guilty for exposing them to pain. While such a wish is understandable, it may not be either realistic or the best preparation for life. Instead of denying that there is a problem, you can demonstrate facing life's challenges and help your children to identify their own feelings. Therapist Geri Ferber, who deals with both infertility and children's issues, feels that there is reason to be concerned about the well-being and the fantasies of children who "accompany their parents on the [infertility] roller coaster."

While the infertility is your crisis, experts agree that it affects your child as well. According to Sharon Jette, former president of and support group leader for RESOLVE of the Bay State, parents can never mask their pain entirely. The stress, the depression, the resentment, and the mood swings that often accompany treatment can "trickle down" to your child.[1] A child's natural inquisitiveness makes hiding the infertility unworkable (even if it were desirable). Pretending that everything is OK and denying your unhappiness are not only confusing to the child but usually unsuccessful. Children can sense when you are preoccupied and not emotionally accessible. If not given an explanation, they rely on their own egocentric perspective and conclude that they are to blame.

The less information available, the more likely children are to resort to fantasy and "magical thinking." Many professionals feel that it is important to address family crises directly to keep children from conjuring up all kinds of strange ideas.[2] Lacking another explanation for unhappiness and doctor's visits, a child might fear that the parent is dying.

What Your Child May Already Know

Pat Johnston, infertility and adoption educator and former chair of the national organization, RESOLVE, Inc., agrees that children often know more than they have been told. In *Taking Charge of Infertility*, she writes:

> Secrets are almost universally impossible to keep. An undercurrent of whispers and overheard bits of conversation, of hesitant or evasive answers to questions, combine to drive children into a fantasy world which can be much more disturbing than reality! Parents walk a tightrope in trying to decide how much is too much and how little is too little, but the overriding thing to remember is that secrets are unhealthy in intimate relationships and can be toxic to family systems.[3]

Even quite young children with whom the infertility had never been overtly discussed have been reported to talk about and even related having had dreams about "the baby" or "my brothers and sisters." While this is a common childhood fantasy, it also seems likely that the children's emotional lightning rods have picked up on this issue.

Regardless of your wishes, practical logistics sometimes dictate how much a child knows about treatment. Parents undergoing treatment involve their children to various extents:

> Our daughter, like many only children, is mature for her age and is very aware of our efforts to conceive. I am undergoing Pergonal treatment, which consumes a great deal of our thoughts, time, and money. My daughter is, of course, aware of all this. She goes with me for daily ultrasounds, helps with shots at home by putting on the Band-Aids, etc. Consequently, she has had to deal with the disappointment of our failures on our first two attempts. We try to keep her from getting her hopes up too much, and she seems to have coped well. Still, I find it difficult to deal with the feeling of letting her down, especially at a time when I feel so disappointed and depressed myself.

If you are using Pergonal or assisted reproductive technologies (ARTs), you know how hard it is to find a babysitter, often at short notice, for the early morning hours when you must have blood drawn, ultrasounds done, or the procedures performed. While it may be possible to call upon a friend or neighbor for a single procedure, most people don't have such resources available on a daily basis.

Most older children receive glimpses into the world of reproduction, some becoming more knowledgeable than many fertile adults. Mothers distressed about this premature introduction to the variations on how babies are made ("How many five-year-olds think women need to take shots to get pregnant?"; "My child thinks that all mommies take their temperature each morning") fantasize that they may be raising future reproductive endocrinologists. One mother explains how her son views reproduction:

> My son does not believe any mammal, including dogs, can reproduce without doctors and having lots of "blood drawn." When told the "facts of life," he told me that is NOT how babies are made. "It takes a doctor and hospital." When I ask my son what he wants to be when he grows up, he says a fireman, after he becomes a doctor and "puts a baby in [my] tummy."

While other children may not possess such specific information, according to Anne Bernstein in *The Flight of the Stork: What Children Think (and When) about Sex and Family Building*, most children believe that "getting babies is a medical enterprise" and the doctor is typically a prominent figure in their accounts of reproduction and birth. She explains that the "belief that medical intervention may be necessary to unite sperm and ovum is one that can occur spontaneously to children, who attribute extraordinary powers to doctors in their attempt to explain aspects of sex and birth that elude their grasp."[4] Cognitively, the medicalization of reproduction may actually make more sense to children that the traditional "facts of life."

What to Tell Your Children

Infertility, because of its very nature, is harder to discuss than other family crises. Determining how much to tell a child and how to do so without shaking his or her basic sense of security presents a challenge for parents. Sharon Jette advocates telling a child about the infertility and resulting sadness and advises parents to "build a vocabulary" with the child to facilitate discussions of loss.[5] Because of your own pain, you may be understandably reluctant to disclose your infertility. Yet children can be wonderfully matter-of-fact about issues that are much more emotionally laden for adults. Some parents project their own feelings of loss onto their children and fear that the children will share their distress and pain. Many children do express the desire for a sibling; while the words may echo your yearning, the emotional weight is not the same.

Often parents worry that children are unable to understand the complexities of infertility. Though this is undoubtably true, "the children aren't looking for a scientific explanation or for a perfectly reasoned thesis. The children simply want to know that everything is okay. . . . [L]ife will go on."[6] According to Rabbi Earl Grollman, who has written extensively on explaining loss to children, parents need not offer more information than the child is really seeking. Some parents overanswer, reflecting their own anxiety, as well as a lack of understanding of their child's cognitive level. Complicated answers create confusion. Most importantly, Grollman advises parents not to tell fairy tales and half-truths. Children need direct, simple, and honest age-appropriate information.[7] *The Flight of the Stork: What Children Think (and When) about Sex and Family Building* by Anne Bernstein explains how children of various ages perceive reproduction. This book is a valuable resource for parents trying to respond to this topic appropriately.

Pat Johnston cautions that parents either fall into the trap cited above of overanswering or else oversimplify to the point of euphemism. She advises that "the more complex the situation, the more important it is to simplify, simplify." She agrees, however, that parents should never give information that is inaccurate resulting in a need to change the story later, for that would compromise trust.[8]

It is fine to tell your child what you believe; however, you must bear in mind that children are cognitively quite literal and may be unable to grasp less concrete and more theological explanations. For instance, following a stillbirth an adult explained to the prospective sibling that "God wanted someone else to have the baby." When new neighbors with a baby moved in, the two-and-a-half-year-old confronted them, saying, "You got my sister!"[9] Similarly, a mother reports that "My three-year-old daughter was told that I 'lost' the baby, and she could not understand why I couldn't find it." It would not be surprising if the child then developed a fear of getting lost herself. A child who is told that "God wanted the baby" might fear that God would want him or her as well.

Care should be taken even when sharing happier news. Some thought should be given before announcing a longed-for pregnancy or adoption, as it is hard for a child to understand a pregnancy loss or an incomplete adoption. Your child might feel that you have broken a promise if things do not work out. Consider the difference to a literal-minded child between saying "We're going to have a baby!" and "We're pregnant." A pregnancy might be likened to a seed that has been planted; not all become flowers. You might wish to convey that while you hope a child will be joining your family through adoption, you cannot guarantee when. Remember that as long as the waiting period seems to adults, it is even longer to children. Some children with no sense of time may expect a sibling immediately.

Pat Johnston specifically discusses how much children should know about their parents' prior infertility. The issues she raises are particularly salient if you are undergoing infertility treatment while parenting small children. The questions are not only more immediate but also more emotionally draining. For instance, in discussing the internal conflicts inherent in parents describing their infertility to their children, she writes,

> Most of the discomfort that nearly all parents have in sharing information about human sexuality with their children comes not from an unwillingness to do this teaching, but instead from their concerns that they won't do it well. *With infertility issues, an additional factor is that the issue that produced the perceived need for information was one which caused the parents a great deal of frustration and pain.* . . . These kinds of internal conflicts—conflicts born of experiences much more sophisticated than any child's—often lead parents . . . to be overly concerned about sharing specifics with children . . . [emphasis added].[10]

What to tell your child about the infertility represents a balancing act. Some parents are quite open with their children about their longing for another child, while preferring to share as little information as possible about the actual treatment, both to protect their children and to maintain their own zone of privacy around such a personal issue. Pat Johnston feels that technical information about reproductive technologies such as IVF or GIFT is too sophisticated for young children to process. Nor does she feel such information is necessary for the child to possess.

One issue in telling a young child is the fear that private information will be broadcast throughout the neighborhood. This has occurred in more than one instance:

> It's hard to explain to a kindergarten-age child why there are no more babies. When I briefly tried to tell him that it was pretty hard for us and that the doctors would help and maybe we'd get a baby someday, he proudly started telling people that Mommy *was* going to have another baby. Off and on for a year, parents, after coming in contact with my confused six-year-old, would congratulate me and ask me when the baby was due.

Another mother who was elated to have a multiple pregnancy and shared this news with her son soon had the painful job of telling her neighbors about her pregnancy loss.

One possible solution, advising your child not to tell, may convey that you are doing something shameful. Children pick up easily on your feelings, and if you feel the infertility is shameful, the child too will perceive it that way. Pat Johnston believes that even young children can understand the need for boundaries; some information is simply private family business. Even so, you may be reluctant to burden your children with information they cannot share. Also, your desire for privacy may raise potentially troubling issues about secrecy; you may not want to establish a precedent for keeping things hidden. As parents, you are the best judges about what will be appropriate for your children, and you may find yourselves being open to a point, while keeping some of the details private.

Another issue unique to this situation is the possibility that your existing child will possess information about the origins of a future sibling. Research is needed to document how such knowledge might affect the child's feelings toward the newcomer if a successful pregnancy or adoption results. Will the future child be less resented and more valued? Will the older child feel that he or she has been a part of the process and feel pride in and a sense of ownership toward a new arrival? Will a future child be blamed for the problems caused and for occupying the parents' attention even before he or she arrived? Will your existing children feel that because you did not go to such lengths to have them, they were less wanted? Will the older child's knowledge determine what is shared in the future? These are difficult questions; however, by considering any possible repercussions in advance, you may prevent potential sibling issues from developing.

How You Can Help Your Child Cope

It is difficult to stand outside your own ongoing crisis and focus on your child's needs. In general, children need to have as much continuity and consistency in their lives as possible. They need to hear that they did nothing wrong; they need to be told that they are loved; they need to know that they will be taken care of; they need to be reassured that you aren't sick; they need to understand enough so that they can maintain trust and not resort to magical thinking; they need to be given permission to verbalize their feelings.

Grieving and Parenting

You may question to what extent your children need reassurance, reasoning that your grief is private and not visible. Following giving birth to a stillborn child, one mother commented, "Jamie was only 2. . . . too young to understand what was happening, which I'm thankful for. It was hard enough coming home with empty arms, let alone trying to explain why to Jamie when I didn't understand why myself."[11] Although this child was too young to ask, that does not necessarily mean that he did not have questions. Sometimes putting comforting thoughts into words is helpful to you and your child alike.

A follow-up study was done on families in which stillbirth occurred which is relevant to families experiencing infertility. This research confirms that even if preschoolers do not understand intellectually, they will pick up on the emotions of an event, knowing that it is a sad moment. A grown-up sibling recalls the loss of a baby sister when he was quite young:

> I remember picking up on the emotions from people around us that something wasn't right. We couldn't play, laugh, or run around. I didn't understand what was really going on, but I remember that feeling.[12]

When sharing a loss with a child, Grollman feels that expressions of the parents' own emotions of grief are appropriate, reasoning that if parents repress their feelings, then children will be more likely to hold their own emotions in check. Parents who mourn give their children a model to follow. While they may feel guilty if they cry in front of their child, Grollman feels that this might actually be a positive act: "It expresses the undeniable fact that you too are human and need emotional release. It is better to say, 'I have been crying [too]' rather than, 'There, there, you mustn't cry.' The most important gift you can give your child is the feeling that life continues despite pain."[13]

The concept of life continuing is a key one for parents. Your children need to be reassured that you will "revive" and that any depression will not be permanent. Further, you can model ways of coping with grief by combining the admission of sadness with constructive examples of what you are doing to alleviate the pain. For instance, "I feel sad, so I talked to a counselor [or friend] about my feelings." It is important that your child feel reassured that although you are dealing with a grown-up problem, someone will always be available to meet his or her needs.

Maintaining Security

Children may be justifiably frightened because it seems as if life will never again be normal and happy. After her mother gave birth to a stillborn child, a daughter asked her father if her mother would ever be happy again.[14] Such a child may try to make everything all right. One four-year-old girl asked her mother, who had miscarried, to curl up into an "S"; she then crawled into the space around her mother's stomach,[15] literally trying to fill the void. Children should not feel responsible for their parents' happiness. While it may be positive for a child to have an opportunity to comfort someone else, children must be secure that grown-ups can take of themselves and them.

Another mother who had experienced pregnancy losses writes, "I'm trying to make his life normal. I don't think at age six he should have an adult burden such as this. . . . I want him to be a happy child, with only childlike concerns." Still, this same mother reports that her son "sees me occasionally with tears and comes over and says he loves me. He asked monthly for the first year, 'Are you going to have a baby yet?' . . . Now he's stopped asking." In this case, the son knew his parents were trying to have a baby, was able to see his mother's cyclic grief, and could share his own feelings of being left out of a school project involving siblings. His mother describes how although her son saw her cry a lot for a year, she tried to be "as normal and consistent as I always was in parenting." It seems that the openness, coupled with consistent childrearing practices showing that his parents still cared about him, provided the basic security this child needed to cope with the sadness around him.

The Role of Others

Support for the child in this as in most crises is often minimal because the focus is on the adults. The parents, hoping that the child is blissfully unaware of their pain, may see no need to help the child sort out his or her own feelings. Caring adults who are not directly involved can be particularly helpful to children during this time, since the child does not feel the need to be careful of their feelings and can therefore express his or her own emotions openly and ask questions without the fear of causing pain.

Relatives, however, may be embarrasssed to hear about infertility, and you may be reluctant to have your child discuss this problem with them. Ideally, other people such as teachers and caregivers should be told about the stress your family is under in order to lend support and interpret any acting-out behaviors. The danger, though, is that such sensitive information might be mishandled and that normal, age-appropriate behavior will be seen as reflecting the stress. It is important for you to avoid blaming your stress for what may be normal developmental issues. Professional advice can be useful if you are concerned about your child's behavior and can also be a source of support for you and your child.

Dealing with Common Concerns

The common childhood fear of something happening to the parents is heightened by the knowledge that the mother or in some cases both parents are undergoing medical treatment. In this case, fantasy and reality converge. Children, like most adults, equate doctors and hospitals with illness. This may be particularly true if your child has witnessed the illness or death of an elderly relative. From their own experiences, children are apprehensive about shots and may be distressed to see you receiving daily Pergonal injections or going to a hospital for ultrasounds. Situations requiring emergency hospitalization, such as ectopic pregnancies, are uniquely trying, since you have no time to prepare for the separation, make arrangements, and provide your child with reassurance.

Some families do have a chance to prepare their child for the mother's upcoming surgery. Carla Harkness quotes one pediatrician who advised a mother to compare her surgery to repairing the car:

> When our car is not working right, we take it to the garage to be fixed by a mechanic who understands about car problems. I have a problem with my body. My doctor, who understands about such things, is going to fix my problem at the hospital. I will be fine and can come home the same day [or in a few days]. I'll have to rest a little more for just a few days [or for a while] after that.[16]

The above narrative may, however, raise some other issues: Is the parent in fact promising that the problem will be fixed? The positive message lies in the reassurance given and the previewing for the child of what will be happening. An added support during a hospitalization would be a calendar or another concrete way in which the child can keep track of how soon the parent will be returning and/or a small gift to open each day from the parent. Some parents tape bedtime stories or messages to their child. The major advantage of scheduled surgery is the opportunity to arrange for consistent childcare and help with driving and other household routines.

Even without hospitalizations, your infertility treatment might cause your child to become fearful:

> Although I try to keep the subject to a bare minimum, I have to explain the doctor visits twice a day when I'm going through a medication cycle. My son gets fearful I'll get sick, because he sees all this medical intervention and he figures if I ever got sick, I'd die, because "the doctors" have not resolved this seemingly simple issue.

Children usually see adults as omnipotent; in this situation, they realize that there are limits to their parents' power and that medical science is not the cure-all that most would like to believe. While the child cited above expresses concerns for his mother, other children may have fears about their own health. It might be useful to explain that while medicine can and does cure most illnesses, there are other grown-up conditions which do not affect children for which doctors do not yet have all the answers. Older children may find even partial medical explanations helpful.

You may feel uncomfortable about being a mother and a patient simultaneously and being forced to consider where to have your child stand during an examination or trying to mask the discomfort of blood tests. Medical staff respond with varying sensitivity to these problems; out of concern for childless patients, some discourage children from being brought to the office, and many mothers share this sensitivity as well. Sometimes, however, it is impossible to avoid taking your child along. Some staff members are willing to distract a child during the crucial treatment or test. One woman relates that her son was so attached to the staff at her doctor's office that he was dismayed when she switched to another medical practice.

At home, many parents try to administer injections privately, after the child is asleep. Your child might question what is going on and why he or she is being excluded. Some parents, however, feel a need to caution their child about the medications and syringes that are stored in the home. Older children have concerns about the use of drugs, having been taught that drugs are "bad," and need to understand that fertility drugs are really medicines prescribed by a doctor.

Children often view events in terms of themselves. Those who have seen their mothers experience a pregnancy loss may become fearful that something will happen to either their mothers or to themselves.[17] One child fantasized that his parents would like to trade him for the child that was lost: "Do you wish we had the other baby rather than me?"[18] While your child may not have any of these reactions, being aware of the possibility of such concerns may enable you to prevent them from arising or to address them if they do.

Children may not express their worries about the parents' infertility and/or unhappiness, because they lack the words, are reluctant to add to the burden, or have received an unspoken message that the subject is off limits, One mother recounts how her daughter developed physical complaints, which she attributes to the stress of the infertility:

> I think [she] couldn't help but feel the stress of our struggles through the medical and adoption mazes. It's a possibility that she uses medical/health problems to get attention when she feels it lacking. Unfortunately, she is very tuned in to me and my every feeling.

Many children do react to changes in the home with physical symptoms. Addressing infertility directly and giving your child permission to express feelings and concerns and to ask questions are ways to prevent or deal with anxiety. Other children may express their anxiety by acting silly, giggling, or being overactive. Such a reaction may seem inappropriate if you don't realize that it reflects discomfort rather than joy.[19]

Addressing Guilt and Magical Thinking

In some cases, normal angry and aggressive wishes will surface as fears if the child tries to hold in all negative feelings. Magical thinking is common; however, children need to be reassured that as Mister Rogers says "wishes don't make things come true."[20] They also need to know that they are not "bad" if they have had angry or even jealous thoughts. Consider the implications in cases of pregnancy loss if the child has harbored normally ambivalent feelings about the prospective sibling. Children who feel that they may have caused a miscarriage either through wishes or by upsetting their pregnant mother may feel that they deserve to be punished for the imagined wrongdoing. Children need to realize that they are not so powerful that their thoughts will prevent conception or cause a loss to occur. Neither will their "being good" make everything all right. Again, the more that you can share, the less likely your child will be to resort to egocentric attributions. For instance, lacking explanations, a child might feel that his parents don't want another child "like him," or, conversely, a child might feel that her parents want another child because of something she has done wrong.

Validating Your Child's Feelings

Some children react to the changes in their parents with anger. One couple report that their son was angered by their fighting caused by infertility-related stresses. Others recall signs of resentment when they "abandoned" their child for surgery or couldn't lift him or her: "I couldn't be the mom she knew, so she would act out or withdraw."[21] Other forms of such perceived abandonment are more subtle, as parents' energy levels are depleted by treatment and depression. (See Chapter 7.) Understanding the reason for your child's behavior and setting aside time to do something pleasurable with him or her can help remedy the situation. It is also positive to acknowledge that the child is angry and to show that you understand and that it is all right to have angry thoughts as long as they are expressed appropriately.

Other children may experience a form of prenatal sibling rivalry. Under these circumstances, they feel displaced by the process of their parents trying to have a baby rather than by a newborn itself. These children, seeing that new babies don't just arrive, may question why their parents want another child so much, feeling that they should be enough.

If you feel your child has emotions that are unexpressed, then creative, free-form activities such as finger paints and fantasy play may allow for expression of his or her mood. Rogers and O'Brien explain that the child uses fantasy to rehearse feelings.[22] This can be a less threatening way for children to express feelings they believe are inappropriate.

Addressing your child's concerns head-on is another way to deal with feelings that may be present but unexpressed. Rogers and O'Brien view open-ended questions as the most effective way to learn what a child is really feeling and to draw out the child's inner thoughts. For instance, "Why do you think Mommy is going to the doctor?" or "How do you feel about having a baby?" If this seems too direct, some experts suggest the use of the third person with young children, for example: "Some children might wonder about . . ." or "Sometimes children might wish. . . ." Psychologist Geri Ferber recommends reading children books about animal characters who experience situations similar to theirs or even helping them to write their own books about imaginary characters. Such conversations should be followed by an invitation for the child to ask questions in order to clear up any misperceptions.

Many parents acknowledge that depression has hindered their ability to cope with their children and have called upon relatives or friends to help out, as discussed in Chapter 7. For example, one woman had a friend care for her child so she could grieve privately. Parenting is demanding work; so is infertility. Infertility treatment is emotionally and physically taxing. As parents dealing with infertility you must deal with your own emotions and your children's at a time when you are most exhausted and drained. As parents, you need to set aside time for yourselves and mobilize as many resources as possible to help you meet your own needs and those of your children. Hopefully, by recognizing the enormousness of your task of nurturing while grieving, you will feel some compassion for yourselves and your situation and reach out to others for the support you and your family need and deserve.

7

Other Parenting Concerns

I'm the only mother my daughter will ever have.
—Mother experiencing secondary infertility

You probably grew up assuming that you would have children.
Not just one child, but rather children in the plural. Although
an increasing number of couples opt for one-child families, it is difficult for many of us to accept a family that differs significantly
from our own family or the family we have fantasized about. The
following accounts reflect the speakers' deep inner conviction that
their families were intended to take a certain form:

> I was always sure that having a family was part of my ultimate happiest
> self, and having a family meant a husband and at least two children.

> I always assumed that I'd have kids, and I think I'd always assumed that
> I'd have three kids; . . . sometimes I think I'm the classic brainwashed
> woman. It was a choice when to have the children, but I never thought
> of not having children. I came from a family of three children, and
> that's why I think I chose that. . . . But to me, a family is three kids be-
> cause that's what I grew up with.

And a father speaks confidently about having a second child:

> There has never been a moment's doubt in my mind from the time I
> had my first child that I would have another and probably another after
> that, so that the idea of having more than one child has always been a
> part of me.[1]

Until couples learn otherwise, most assume that they can choose
their desired family size. When this goal is frustrated, it is necessary
to try to reconcile your expected with your existing family. Parenting

91

a single child may be very different from the way in which you were raised. Secondary infertility brings up feelings about your own family, your siblings, and what constitutes a "real" family.

The Ideal Family

Infertile couples all grapple with their ideas of what makes a family: Does being a family require children, and if so, how many? While on some level couples know that they and a single child are a family, it may not always feel like what a "REAL FAMILY" should be. As the adoptive mother of a second child put it, yes, one child does make a family, but "two is *more* of a family." It's hard to define what makes a family:

> We have a child, but we won't have a family until we have a child to share with our daughter or I change my mind about what a family is. In my heart, I know we're a family, and I try to concentrate on that and all the positives. However, it's not always possible. Sometimes I just cry and try to get it out of my system.

A smaller family than expected can raise issues of boundaries between parent and child and challenge your sense of completeness:

> I have never felt complete with a family of three (one child) and have always wondered how my perception of a "complete family" affects my daughter. We try to always invite another child or two to join us wherever we go. Just hanging around the house seems incomplete without more children for Beth to play with. There is always a sense of imbalance when the three of us are together. Beth struggles for adult attention, and seems to feel left out when my husband and I are conversing.

One man sees siblings as necessary in order to establish clear boundaries:

> Well, I think as a matter of principle kids should have siblings. I think that instead of a family in which there's the king, queen and the prince, it's much better to have the kids versus the parents. That way the kids have allies and have to learn to deal with their peers. There was sibling rivalry in my family, but there was also a lot of kids teaming up against the parents. The kids formed their own society. . . . We had long fantasies, worlds that we created that our parents weren't part of.[2]

Questioning the legitimacy of your family can cause feelings of failure and even lead to acute distress:

> I looked at my handsome husband, and thought about the beautiful children he could have had with someone else. I wanted to die, so that he could have children with another wife, and give our daughter siblings. I contemplated suicide. Somehow, I couldn't feel like we were a true, legitimate family.

The inability to achieve your desired family can cause you to mourn for your intended children, who may have been visualized in great detail:

> Our ideal family has two kids—a blond, curly haired, funny little girl who dances and sings and a little dark-haired boy who collects things and loves history like his dad—but the little boy is in our dreams and prayers.

Just as attention has been paid to the mesh between parent's and child's personalities, so too do I propose that there is also a mesh between parenting style and family personality. Some parents might prefer to focus on one child at a time or might feel less harassed parenting one child. Others, however, crave the interaction of siblings and cannot visualize parenting a single child:

> After much thought I feel it boils down to my sense of family . . . life was noisy, the phone was busy. . . . Parents were peripheral. It's the commotion that I always wanted—enough to give me that slightly distracted look, that amazingly selective deaf ear, that automatic swaying motion. . . . Now things are clean, neat. But I don't want it all tidy or quiet or organized! I want shrieks of laughter, frogs in a drawer or two, ballgames in the yard, a constant search for the other shoe.[3]

Some feel more comfortable parenting more than one child:

> One child felt too enmeshing. I was too overidentified with my first child; I felt like I was burdening him too much with my issues. Having our second child was . . . a way of helping me to disengage myself from overinvolvement with Seth. Now there's a clearer sense of the separateness between my children and me.[4]

Another woman, fearing she would be overprotective, reasoned that three children would be ideal for her, since her involvement would be diluted and, out of necessity, she would have to let go.

Feelings about Own Family

Most people base their image of family on a replication of or a re-action to the family in which they grew up. For instance, one woman expected that she too would have a large family and regrets that her daughter will lack that experience:

> As one of five kids I grew up in a . . . community where it seemed everyone did things in multiples of five: the Smiths had five, the Jones had ten, was it the Maloneys or the Dugans with fifteen? . . .
>
> I always wanted not fifteen, and maybe not even five, but enough. . . . To this end . . . I found a husband who I knew would be a good father. I chose a profession that allowed me to set up a home office. We designed and built a house with multiple bedrooms for use, not show.
>
> Will our daughter ever know the mischief of sisters caught with Mom's makeup, the frustration of having to share her toys (or clothes) all the time, the confidences which can't bridge generations? And when we get old and start acting funny, who will she call and say, "We've got to get Mom to stop wearing T-shirts to Garfinkel's." . . . I want her to have buddies, who for half of her life she'll probably think are truly foreign but, in the end, they are family and they'll always be there.[5]

While some people need to replicate the size of their own family, others identify with their own birth position. Adult and child psychiatrist Miriam Mazor, M.D. recounts the poignant remark of a patient experiencing secondary infertility who had been a second child herself: "The child we didn't have was me."

In another case, a large age gap within her spouse's family provides an acceptable alternative to a woman's own closely spaced siblings:

> I used to cry and cry that my boy was getting older and he'd never have a close sibling. When he was three or four, and family members were having their second and third children, it was so hard for me. Now that he's nine, I try to think of all the good that will come out of the spread in ages and concentrate on that part of the sibling relationship he might still have. Thank God my husband is fourteen years older than his youngest sister because I have clung to their relationship as proof that there will still be some of the closeness I feel for my four brothers and sisters, who, along with me, were born over a short, nine-year span and were very close in age.

Sometimes family relationships that are viewed realistically as less than ideal still determine the script for what a family should be:

> Although I don't necessarily like my husband's family, on the holidays when we do get together, it is nice to have such a large get-together. Together we have ten nieces and nephews! . . . One child just doesn't seem right to me.

Others consciously decide to establish a family that differs from their own, only to find that this is not possible:

> I came from a very large Catholic family and wanted to raise two kids in a relatively peaceful environment—different from the noise and chaos I knew from my upbringing. We spent a lot of time talking about the merits of having two vs. three children.

Similarly, another woman, who was one of ten children, wanted to have two children so that each would feel special; however, the idea of having a child with no siblings was completely alien. Sometimes a less-than-ideal sibling relationship can minimize the tendency to idealize the big happy family:

> I grew up with two older sisters and was never close to them; in fact, the three of us practically fought and competed against each other our whole life, and to this day, we are not close. I've often told my mother, "It did me no good to have two siblings—we are not close at all—so perhaps Julia is better off not having siblings." When she is lonely for friends, we just invite them over to play.

Another woman who didn't get along with her sister remarks that she "sometimes feels a sibling is a nasty trick to play on your child"; however, she explains, she wants another child not for her daughter, but rather for her own sake.

Others strive to create for their child the supposedly ideal family they lacked in their own life. Parents, despite or perhaps because of the reality of their own sibling relationships, tend to view having siblings as more beneficial than "onlyship."[6] Psychiatrist Miriam Mazor M.D. explains that often those who have been disappointed in their relationship with their own brothers and sisters hope to provide their children with the ideal relationship they themselves lacked.[7] Infertility tends to accentuate this normal developmental response.

While many adults who were single children prefer that their own children have siblings, this is not universal. Those who in childhood were lonely, identified too much with adults, or grew up too soon fear that their child will have the same problems. Or they may feel the need to compensate for the perceived deprivations of their childhood by creating the "big happy family" they longed for themselves as a child:

> I grew up as an "only child." I begged and cried and cried for brothers and sisters, especially sisters, but then my mother and dad got a divorce. . . . I grew up, even then, envious and jealous of big happy families. I always wanted bunkbeds like everyone else but never had need for them. My favorite television shows were "The Waltons" and "Little House on the Prairie." How I dreamed someday I could create my own family, surrounded by the blessings of children and the closeness of family to make up for my lonely childhood.

Some parents can differentiate between their experiences as a single child and those of their children, who may have different personalities and life circumstances:

> I was an "only" child for ten years before my brother was born. I was lonely. I was also shy—my son is not. There were adults all around, and I felt I grew up faster—always communicated on an adult level. I see that aspect in my son—he communicates like an adult. But I've always encouraged him to play with friends, and he has two boys he's close with in our neighborhood.

Other adults who themselves had no siblings can appreciate the advantages of having been the only child and feel unprepared to deal with sibling conflicts. One woman whose husband is a single child sees "great benefits in that, as well as in having siblings."

You might also have specific concerns based on your own backgrounds. Those with aging parents know firsthand the advantages of sharing responsibilities with siblings:

> It really never occurred to me to have only one child; it sounds so lonely to me. Also, my father died almost twelve years ago, and when I look at my semiaging mother, . . . I am glad that I won't have to make the decisions regarding her alone, as I have an older brother and a younger sister.

Your own personal circumstances can also influence your ideas about what a family should be. For instance, older parents fear that their children will be left alone once they are gone.

> Much of my concern focuses on my daughter. I worry about her being lonesome and alone. Fortunately, she is wonderful at entertaining herself and playing by herself, which is great. She is also a very happy and balanced child. But since she is the only child of older parents, she is likely to have to be on her own before most kids, and before I would like her to be.

Weighing the Importance of the Sibling Relationship

While many experiencing secondary infertility already have more than one child, for those who don't, the desire to provide a sibling for the existing child is a frequent and powerful motivation. This desire not only grows from internal forces, such as fantasies about the ideal family and reactions to one's own family, but also is shaped by outside forces, such as public opinion about the desirability of siblings and the stigma that is still attached to being or having a so called "only child."

The Needs of the Existing Child

While women with primary infertility commonly express regrets about failing their husbands as wives by not reproducing, women with secondary infertility more often state that they are failing their children as mothers by not providing them with siblings. Parents want what is best for their child, and many experts cite the advantages of the sibling relationship. For instance, Lee Salk, M.D. states that "sibling attachments can be among the strongest and most rewarding over a lifetime."[8] Parents respond not only to such expert opinion but also to their own perceptions about families. For instance, the woman quoted below feels guilty since she believes that being an only child is hard:

> Secondary infertility adds a new source of guilt—I felt I had let my son down! I had always believed that it is hard on a child to grow up being an only child and that his development would be better if he had brothers and sisters. Not only did I have a dim view of myself because I

couldn't conceive, but I thought that I couldn't do what was best for the son I did have by providing brothers and sisters.[9]

In addition to expert advice and your own feelings, you may be besieged by pleas from your child for a sibling. For some, the sense of failing their child is the most difficult part of secondary infertility. As one woman stated, "Most of all, I felt for my only child, who wanted a sibling desperately." Another woman relates her son's confusion and sadness:

> When you have one child and can't have another, not only do you have to struggle with your and your husband's frustration, guilt, and sadness; now you have to add a little boy that wants brothers and sisters like everyone else in his world. It's hard to explain to a kindergarten-age child why there are no more babies.

It is quite possible that children pick up on the societal norm for families and realize that their family is somehow different. Today big happy families like the "Brady Bunch" and the "Partridge Family" continue to dominate the airwaves via cable and have been supplemented by programs idealizing contemporary forms of such families—for instance, "Full House," in which a main character explicitly states that he was an only child and now enjoys being part of a "family." It is painful to feel that your child is being set apart or deprived. One woman recalls how her daughter went for a walk with her aunt and her new baby. She came back proudly talking about "how anyone driving by might think she was part of a real family." Another describes how her nine-year-old son is "very aware that he is an only child":

> He is the only one in his class without siblings. His friends ask him why he doesn't have brothers and sisters. He feels left out of conversations when other kids talk about their siblings.
>
> Too many times after being around babies he will ask me, "When are we going to have a brother or sister?" It hurts me when I see him this way, and it hurts even more when I think I may not be able to give him what he so badly wants.[10]

Other Motivations for Wanting Another Child

You may want to have another child in part so that your existing child will not be lonely, assuming that siblings will be playmates and companions. One at-home mother describes the difficulty of being a playmate for her child and longs for another child to fill this role. Increasingly, children today are attending daycare and obtaining companionship and peer socialization from that contact. Yet, while other social experiences can alleviate loneliness, parents often have special expectations of the sibling relationship. A book on sibling relationships details this perspective:

> Parents often fantasize that their children will magically become close, affectionate, and mutually responsive and may even remain life-long friends—a parental legacy expressed in the phrase "after we're gone, you'll always have each other. . . ." Such fantasies can be compensatory, stemming from either parent's memories of his or her own painful sibling experiences in childhood. For many parents, regardless of their histories, envisioning a close and cozy set of siblings fulfills their ideal of the "perfect" family.[11]

While there is certainly some merit to this view, the reality is considerably more complex, as has been discussed. One note of caution: As parents who are striving to have another child, you may tend to idealize the sibling relationship both to yourselves and to your children. It may then be a source of disappointment to the older children if a baby does arrive through birth or adoption to find out that, no matter how badly wanted, a baby is just that—a baby!

According to T. Berry Brazelton, M.D. parents are usually motivated to have another child by a combination of factors. They may feel that one child will be too lonely if both parents are working or fear that an only child may be "spoiled" or may "suffer." Some feel that they should have a second child in order to give the first a friend and a close relative. A less conscious motivation may be the desire to have a child for each parent. One woman verbalizes this wish: "A little girl to be 'me' and a little boy to be 'him.'" Brazelton confirms that many families today have two children as their goal.[12]

Despite the forces promoting families with more than one child, single-child families may be the most rapidly growing family form. It has been reported that more than 20 percent of married couples in the United States have one child. This trend is growing, due to the economy and the expense of childrearing and the fact that more couples are delaying childbearing and are reluctant because of age to have anymore. These couples may also understand the difficulties of childrearing and decide that one is all they can handle.[13] While this explanation does not take secondary infertility into account, it provides a context for understanding why couples might choose to have one. This rationale is of little comfort when you do want to have additional children; however, the demographic shift should begin to lessen the stigma of being or having a single child.

Merle Bombardieri, author of *The Baby Decision* and an infertility therapist, believes that the only good reason to have another child is the strong desire for one. She cites common motivations that she feels are not sufficient reasons, such as the first child becoming too grown-up, the need for a change or to provide meaning to your life, the pressure of others, the myths about onlies, the desire for a child of another sex, or as a companion for the existing child. She points out that there is no guarantee that siblings would enjoy each other's company and that it is "much easier to arrange a social life for the first" than to have another child to provide companionship.[14]

Parents may not always be conscious of their motivation for wanting another child; it may be that on a fundamental level, their family just does not feel complete as it is. Some women have powerful images of what a family should be; one woman visualized filling up the backseat of her car and having a child to sit in the extra chair at her table. Others describe families with more children as looking "right" or report that they feel better when they take an additional child along on an outing.

Concerns about Spacing Children

Not only are "good parents" supposed to provide siblings for their child, but there is also a presumably correct way to space them for optimal development. Actually, there are advantages and disadvantages to all forms of spacing, just as there are to having siblings at all. There is more diversity in today's families than there has been in the recent past, such as the 1950s. Some blended families incorporate the children of two marriages, who may vary greatly in age. Other couples delay childbearing, then have children in rapid succession or decide to stop at one. And as you well know, other couples find that, contrary to popular opinion, not all families can be planned. Still, the idea of proper spacing intensifies the perceived time pressure to conceive:

> Time is so marked as your first child ages and you start to calculate what the age difference will be.
>
> Although at thirty-four I still have a number of years left in which I could, theoretically, get pregnant, I feel that my daughter's quickly getting past the age of having a sibling relationship. Even if my current attempt succeeds, she will already have turned eight before I have another baby.

While you may have a preferred spacing for your children in mind, clearly there are pros and cons to parenting children who are close together in age. Whole books have been written debating the advantages and disadvantages, and experts do not always agree. Siblings close in age share more activities and life events; however, they may also "collide and struggle" with one another more frequently.[15]

Just because you did not choose to space siblings in a certain way does not mean that there aren't advantages to it. Brazelton cites many benefits to spacing children more than three years apart, even telling of pregnant mothers who break down, feeling they are abandoning their first child. He quotes Margaret Mead as lamenting that in our culture, children four to seven years old rarely have the opportunity to care for smaller children. There is also believed to be an intellectual advantage in spacing children several years apart. Above all, Brazleton feels that spacing should be a "selfish decision,"[16] reasoning that if parents are happy with the spacing, the older child will adjust to any configuration. This reasoning may hold for children without siblings as well.

Attitudes toward Single Children

You may be motivated not only by your own wishes and the desire to do what you consider best for your child but also by the perceived need to avoid the stigma of having an "only child." In fact, the phrase "only child" has become so negative that I prefer to speak in terms of a "single child." One mother rejects applying this label to her family:

> I think of our family as my "dream family" in terms of more than the current three. People refer to my boy as an only child, and I hate that term. I tell people, "He's my only child right now, but he won't be forever."

The popularly held view is that "only children" are somehow at emotional risk, even though research has documented many positives that correspond to being a single child, such as high achievement, high self-esteem, and academic and occupational success. A study of only children has confirmed that these children have had a negative image, but points out that such stereotypes as the only child as "selfish, handicapped, anxious, not fun to be with, egotistical, [and] at a disadvantage when it comes to making his own way in a world" are "long on myth, short on actual research."[17] (See Chapter 9, "Considering Possible Outcomes.")

Currently, this negative view remains so pervasive that parents are blamed for having only one child. The behavior of a single child is often scrutinized by others for signs of stereotypical "only" behavior. It may be that other parents, feeling overwhelmed by the demands of their children, need to bolster their own decision to have more than one by finding fault with "onlies." Teachers and school personnel are not immune to this prejudice, and even playmates can call an only child spoiled.

You may have internalized this view yourself, falling victim to the same myths. For instance, some parents worry about a child who is clingy, has difficulty separating at daycare or school, or is demanding, fearing that such normal developmental behaviors are due to the child's being an "only." While some parents attribute such behavior to being an "only child," other parents are rethinking these stereotypes:

> My current perception of only children is positive in some respects. It seems environmentally "correct" and as though the child has more of a chance at getting quality attention. In our case, we are surrounded by so much family and friends that being lonely is not one of our concerns for our child. My old perception is that only children are lonely and spoiled. However, I cannot think of anyone I know that falls into the latter category that is an only child.

Such reality checking is useful; it can validate your success in raising a well-adjusted single child and enable you to appreciate some of the positives. As one mother comments,

Before I *had* an only child, I felt that most are doted on, spoiled, etc. But my eleven-year-old son seems to be pretty well adjusted. He is protective of some of his things, but shares, is thoughtful of others, has a good sense of humor, and is good company. I really like that I have the time and money (the luxury) to provide him with piano lessons, books, outings, *and* to enjoy these things with him.

Sometimes confronting your fears about parenting an only child is the best way to combat them. One woman did so with the help of a therapist:

Before I entered therapy, I was upset at the thought of my son being an only, but the therapist soon made me realize that it totally depends on the parenting. I think there is a stigma attached to being an only. There is a stereotype of the spoiled, self-centered child, but my son doesn't fit that mold at all.

Experts speak of trade-offs between child "quantity and quality." Some parents actively research this topic and are pleased with what they learn:

I think only children are great. I read a lot about them in preparation. They are very smart—many are astronauts. Miss America '93 is one. I was always impressed with the attention they get from their parents. They do not have to compete with other siblings.

Some parents see advantages to their child being raised as a single child, but have concerns about their child being alone in later life:

My feelings about only children are mixed. I do not believe that only necessarily means lonely; nor do I feel that only children are necessarily selfish. I believe that only children may have a very positive advantage in that they are given full support and attention from both parents, which can be a very positive influence in all that they do. My worries are more for the future, when my husband and I are older or gone. I feel a lot of support as an adult from my siblings, and it is difficult for me to imagine what it would be like without this support.

Strategies for parenting a single child that address these concerns are presented later in this chapter.

Impact of Infertility on Parenting

Parenting the single child shares some of the same dynamics as parenting after infertility as described in *The Long-Awaited Stork: A Guide to Parenting after Infertility* by Ellen Glazer. Many parents experiencing secondary infertility are parenting single children. Some are also parenting after prior infertility. But all are parenting during infertility. This combination of factors is potentially loaded, and parents commonly report being overprotective or fearful about the existing child, as well as feeling ambivalent about developmental advances that might otherwise be an occasion for joy. As parents mourn for the children they may never have, they may also be acutely aware that they will never have another chance to enjoy the child they do have. The following vignette touches on many common themes in parenting during infertility—the pain and feelings of failure at depriving your child of a sibling, the poignancy of each stage of development, the tendency to be overprotective and not let go, and the bittersweet feelings about parenthood:

> Katie has wanted to go out and buy a baby. A friend was over and said that they were having a new baby. Katie said, "We're not having a baby." It felt like a knife in the heart.
>
> I'm also very protective of Katie. I worry about her a lot. I always think that she's the only child I have and [that I] may only have her. . . .
>
> At times, I feel like selling all the baby stuff because it's a constant reminder of the baby we've been trying to have. . . . Every time I look at my daughter, I remember my pregnancy, her birth, her first three months of colic when I would have given her away if she weren't so cute, her being an infant, a toddler, . . . her emergence as a preschooler. I know she doesn't need me like she once did, but I want her to go to school and be secure—so I'll be brave and send her off with a kiss and a hug and pray that she'll do fine on her own. . . .
>
> I feel like a failure for not providing my child with a sibling. I feel like I'm depriving her of something.

Overprotectiveness and Extra Attention

Infertile parents tend to focus much attention on their existing child or children, and doing so has the potential for both positive and negative results. As one parent says, both parents may "focus too much on that child, and everything . . . is magnified—the good and the bad." Another parent explains that because of her need to parent more children, she "focused excess energy on parenting my daughter, thus simultaneously indulging and demanding from her." One mother describes how she worked to establish some balance in her relationship with her son:

> There have been times that my feelings (sadness, frustration, depression) affected my interactions with my son. Sometimes I felt I had no energy for him. At other times the focus on him became too much, too intense. Something like, "Since I only have one child, you have to be perfect." But establishing a good balance with him has evolved as I've become more "normal" about this. I was worried that he'd feel he wasn't enough or wasn't good enough, and I've talked with him about it.

The knowledge that losses occur can create fear, which may lead to overprotectiveness but also to cherishing the existing child:

> It's hard not to be overprotective, because I now know how really irreplaceable children are. . . . I feel like my innocence has ended, and I know now that "bad things can happen to good people." I feel like if I love my husband and little boy too much, they'll be the next to get hit by the erring semitruck—as if tragedy can hone in on you like a heat-seeking missile if you are vibrating too much love. Both my husband and I baby our boy; we read or talk to him until he goes to sleep every night and sometimes don't wake up to stumble into our own bed. It's as if, if we can see him, he's OK.

Children may, however, remain unaffected by their parents' concern: "I feel I have become a little bit obsessive about my son—especially in regard to health issues. But my feelings have fortunately not rubbed off on him, due to his personality." Another mother is "mildly concerned" about the potential for her daughter to be "overprotected or smothered." Your awareness of this possibility may be the surest way to prevent it. The fallout from infertility is not entirely negative: "On the positive side, we cherish every day with our son. We know how precious his childhood days are. On the downside, we are probably overprotective in letting him take risks."

Ambivalence about Children's Growth

By the time you recognize and begin treatment for an infertility problem, your first child may have started nursery school or even elementary school and may no longer be as dependent on you. This is frequently a trying time for all parents, even those who have not experienced infertility. The following describes the typical reactions of such mothers to their children growing up:

> Each step in a child's development that makes a mother feel proud can also make her feel hurt and rejected when she realizes that her child does not need her in the way he or she once did. For example, "Mommy, me do it!" I was crushed . . . because I realized that the time is going by so quickly.

Sending a child off to school can be a pivotal point because the child becomes a part of a larger world: "But then the bus came, . . . and it hit me that she was entering a new world, a world that for much of her day would not include me. I cried the whole day."[18]

For those who have been unable to have other children, every developmental step is particularly poignant: greeted with pride, but also with the realization that this stage will not come again. Even subtle markers of growth, such as the desire for privacy or the reluctance to cuddle, can become emotionally charged milestones. A normal desire of a child to separate and gain autonomy can be especially painful if the parents are experiencing the "empty lap" syndrome.

You may be concerned about holding on to your child and not letting her or him grow up. One mother who had a son following primary infertility and was unable to have additional children made a point of celebrating each advance in her son's development as a deliberate strategy to counter her own ambivalent feelings.[19]

Being unable to have another child can make it harder to let go of your existing child, who may be needed to fill a void. One mother who had experienced a pregnancy loss describes that dynamic: "I had encouraged her independence during my pregnancy, but after the loss of the baby, I needed to be needed by her." Another mother explains that while she was pregnant, she encouraged her firstborn to be a "big girl," and once she miscarried, she recast her as her baby. It is not possible for one child to compensate for your loss of another. A child no matter how loved, cannot take the place of a baby: "Our 2 + year old daughter has truly been a comfort to me, but still no matter how tightly I hold her in my arms, I feel an emptiness that she cannot fill."[20]

Loss of Mother Role

For mothers experiencing infertility, and fathers perhaps to a lesser extent, the infertility represents not only the loss of the longed-for child but also the inability to perpetuate the mothering role, which may have been central to their identity and daily existence. Social worker Karen Berkeley, observes that "as their child[ren] grows out of toddlerhood, they often panic at the thought of never having another baby."[21]

Typically, whether or not they've worked outside the home, mothers struggling to have another child have invested a great deal in parenting. Some have deferred career advancement to parent; many have juggled the demands of family, job, and infertility treatment; and all share a commitment to parenting. It seems unfair to many of them that they are being deprived of another child when less deserving or even abusive women seem to have all the children (or even more than) they want. Sometimes parents try to be what they consider to be ideal parents, hoping to prove themselves worthy of a pregnancy or adoption. But, another child is not a reward for good parenting; nor is infertility a judgment of unfitness.

In some cases, parents have a desire to have another child so that they can "get it right the second time." Normal regrets about their parenting are intensified, since they won't have a chance to learn from their mistakes and build on their experience. Also, just as the single child may feel a need to be perfect, parents who sense that this may be their only chance at parenting may feel required not only to "do it all" but also to be unambivalently enthusiastic about their parenting duties.

Many women have a desire not only to have another child but also to reexperience pregnancy, childbirth, and nursing. These may have been peak experiences for a woman, a time during which she felt special, and she yearns to recapture those feelings. One woman analyzes the impact of her pregnancy and birthing experiences on her desire to give birth again:

We had a great birth experience and wanted more of the same. My desire goes deeper than my husband's, though. Mine has been a longing that is partly fueled by the experience of pregnancy. I have a physical yearning for it.

Others regret that they did not focus on these experiences the first time, not realizing that they would not be repeated:

I wanted to be pregnant and experience the miracle of giving birth again. I really wanted to have a baby to nurse. I wanted to pay attention this time and appreciate the details. My son's babyhood, toddlerhood, flew by me somehow. I felt I'd missed it.

On the other hand, parents who have conceived their first child through ARTs and want more children must decide how long they will wait before re-entering treatment, if treatment is again indicated. They must weigh their desire to enjoy the child they have against their concern that the likelihood of having another child will decrease with time. Experiencing the babyhood of their longed for child is particularly poignant when they are already questioning whether or not they will ever pass this way again.

Bittersweet Experience of Parenting

Ironically, your very joy in parenting can underscore the pain of your infertility. You cannot pretend to be child-free or convince yourself that parenting might not be so great after all. You know all about parenting and opted for more children. The paradox is that the more positive you feel about your existing child, the more pain you may experience if you are unable to have another. One woman writes, following a hysterectomy,

I'm left with this absolutely gorgeous, smart, active two-year-old who is driving me crazy because she is everything I can't have. . . . She is the dream of my unborn children. I love her tremendously, but that is what makes my unborn children seem so unjustified.

In the same vein, another mother laments, "Our daughter is such a blessing to us, more than I could ever say. That is why we so desperately want more, a sister or brother for her and an opportunity for us to have a bigger family."

Unfortunately, some parents find that their mixed emotions make it hard for them to enjoy the children they do have. Your child can become a constant and painful reminder of the longed-for children. Older children, no matter how loved, do not take the place of another child; nor should they. They must be appreciated for themselves. Some parents, depressed by their infertility, temporarily experience a loss of interest in the existing child; this has the potential to compound their loss. One mother describes her ambivalent emotions: "Sometimes I felt it was difficult to be around him; sometimes it was hard to let go of him and let him grow up." Another mother felt that due to depression, she was only "going through the motions of parenting."

Karen Berkeley, a support group leader for RESOLVE of the Bay State, cautions that the child who is there will never be any younger and that parents who cannot enjoy the children as they mature may experience regret later.[22] The dilemma becomes how much energy to devote to pursuing a pregnancy as opposed to investing in the child already there. Berkeley states the problem, "Involvement, and in some cases obsession, with medical treatment or natural attempts at pregnancy can eclipse the joy and poignancy of the present moment with the child they do have."[23]

Parenting under Stress

A common concern expressed by mothers is the difficulty in remaining a good parent while undergoing the stress of treatment and medications:

> Treatment creates stress—but you can't walk away from your family to deal with it whenever you might like. It is so hard to cope, grieve, scream—*and* parent. I also sometimes think—and deeply regret—that I have "lost" my daughter's youngest years, because often I was so immersed in the pain and grief of infertility. I worried that we made her feel inadequate because we had to try so hard to have another child.

> While I was on fertility drugs that worsened my depression, there were times that I was emotionally out of control. At these times, parenting was very difficult. I had little patience or tolerance for my son. Luckily, my husband and my parents were available to step in and help.

The awareness that treatment is compromising their ability to parent causes some parents to discontinue treatment: "All the emotion from the treatment, as well as the emotions from the hormones, made it very difficult not to be angry and frustrated much of the time. It is one of the biggest reasons we discontinued treatment."

A lack of patience is a frequent complaint, often compared with having an ongoing "healthy case of PMS." As one mother worried,

> I feel I have much less patience for my daughter, and then I feel guilty about it. I snap at her for little things, and I'm afraid she'll grow up hating me or thinking I'm nuts.

Another woman expresses her distress about the past and its potential effects on her son:

> I wonder if my emotional state of the past may have had an effect on our son. As my work-up was proceeding, I became more depressed and drawn into myself. I became extremely overprotective of our son. I was terrified that something would happen to him. I couldn't bear the thought of losing him and watched over him constantly. I knew he had to venture out on his own, but I resisted each new step in his life that he had to take. I am sure that the hardest time for him was when I was depressed and cried all the time. How could he understand what was happening when I didn't understand it? I am not so sure that he didn't blame himself for some of my moods. Today I try to make it clear to him that it is not his fault. Sometimes I am fearful that my emotional state in the past may have caused problems with our son that will surface in the future.[24]

The following account describes the impact of his mother's prolonged depression and his father's emotional distance on a five-year-old. His mother was able to turn the situation around by seeking counseling and support. When the five-year-old "made a fuss about everything" and "cried with no explanation," the mother consulted a priest:

> My priest helped me to realize that I was paying more time and attention to the babies who died than to the child I had. This helped me to start to accept the losses more. I started to feel so grateful for my son. Afterward I noticed a change in Warren. He got better after I changed toward him.[25]

On the other hand, some parents feel that their parenting has not been affected or has only changed for the better:

My ability to parent has not changed through infertility. I have some short-tempered or sad days at times, but I believe that all parents have these types of days with their children. My relationship to my son may be changed a little in that I now try to enjoy each stage that he goes through as a mother may try to enjoy the stages of a child that she knows will be her last.

Because I realize how blessed I am to have him, I try not to take him for granted. I take advantage of the fact that I can give him my undivided attention. I try to be patient with him and savor his childhood. When I get frustrated with him, I try to remind myself how lucky I am to have him, and I try to be more tolerant.

Still others, aware of the difficulties, try to do their best for their children despite the pressures:

I will try very, very hard to not let it affect my daughter. I remind myself that I am living for her—she needs me to be alive and loving and caring. She needs her mother, and . . . I need to live, fully and happily.

Some parents who have experienced pregnancy losses find that caring for a surviving child helps you as much as it helps the child, since the child's love and need for you "reaffirm your role as a parent." One suggests planning with your child some special activities that can help both of you heal emotionally.[26] Another mother agrees, realizing that although she is depressed because her daughter may be her only child, she will definitely be her daughter's only mother, and as such has a vital role to play in her development.

It can be difficult during infertility to help your child socialize with peers who may have pregnant mothers and infant siblings. (See Chapter 5, "Caught between Two Worlds.") Taking a child to nursery school has been described as traumatic, since all the other mothers had infants with them or were pregnant. One mother explains:

I used to *dread* playground, playgroup, and preschool activities because one or two of the other moms was always pregnant—often with number three or four!

To some extent, this problem may be a function of your child's age; older children are both more independent and less likely to have friends whose mothers are having babies. Most parents acknowledge two things: the difficulty of participating in such activities and the need to do so for their children's sakes. Many continue to attend despite the difficulty, because the child needs the "consistency, enjoyment, and socialization," and they are reluctant to deprive the child "because it's hard to look at babies."

Strategies for Parenting a Single Child

The way parents feel about having a single child and whether this is the result of "choice or fate" can be key in how that child is reared. Those who have chosen to have a single child may feel no need to compensate for any perceived deprivation and may be more relaxed and accepting. On the other hand,

> [p]arents who would like to have several children but who can have only one seem prone to load some of their disappointment on the only child and to create in that child special problems. . . . A classic message that disappointed parents pass on to the only child is this: "You're all we've got, and, by God, you'd better be everything to us all of the time."[27]

This needn't be the case, however. Peg Beck, a clinical social worker and director of RESOLVE of the Bay State, conducts workshops for parents entitled "Stopping at One: Considering a Family of Three" in which she suggests strategies for parenting single children. These include validating that families come in all shapes and sizes, expressing both positive feelings and regrets about the family, letting friends become family and family become friends, and asking for support. Further, she points out the particular importance of parents getting along with each other so that the child is not pulled into a triangle. Some specific recommendations are sharing vacations with families with children, establishing "mutual childcare," keeping family journals and photo albums to provide remembrances and continuity for the child in later life, and planning ahead for your future needs if you become ill so that your child is not responsible for making decisions alone. Above all, positive relationships within the existing family can be the most important factor for your child.

It is important to be aware of the potential pitfalls in parenting during the stresses of infertility, and to try to enlist additional support for yourselves and your children. (Specific suggestions on helping your child cope with the infertility are discussed in Chapter 5.)

Karen Berkeley suggests that parents make a conscious effort to treasure and enjoy this time with their children. Though many situations bring secondary infertility into "sharp and painful relief, they are also precious and irretrievable moments for you and your child. There are myriad opportunities to create lasting memories."[28]

III

Possible Resolutions to and Strategies for Coping with Secondary Infertility

8

Working with Your Medical Providers

The days of 'doctor as God' are over.
—Isaac Schiff, M.D.

While you may have an excellent relationship with your health care team, for others the emotional crisis of secondary infertility may be exacerbated by confusion, delays, or even mistakes in medical treatment. Medical decision making for secondary infertility can be complicated by assumptions based on past fertility. While medical protocols in the treatment of primary infertility appear to be somewhat standardized, many doctors are slower to treat cases of secondary infertility. You may have been relieved to be advised to follow a low-key approach—at least at first.

Seeking Treatment

If you had a good relationship with your OB/GYN, this is probably where you began diagnosis and treatment. For some, the prior relationship presents an obstacle, and they report difficulty in "trying to convince the OB/GYN who delivered your child that you are having an infertility problem." Returning to a place with happy memories while confronting a new issue can drive home your change in status:

It was difficult to return to the doctor and clinic where I had gone when pregnant. It had been reassuring then to see Carl Saunders's quote "A baby is God's opinion that life should go on," but the memory of that

117

stung as I sat in the waiting room. Before, I was part of the happy group of pregnant women, looking through magazines while waiting my turn; now, I wanted to hide from them, not wanting to face what I so desperately wanted but couldn't have.

If you had prior infertility, you may be aware of other resources; however, those of you with first-time infertility may have no idea where to turn or even be aware that specialized care for your problem exists. Many people do not even realize that secondary infertility is possible. A typical problem for both you and your doctor is the tendency to make assumptions based on prior fertility or successful infertility treatments. According to Diane Clapp, medical director of RESOLVE, Inc., "Oftentimes the medical community and Ob/Gyn generalists dismiss secondary infertility. . . . Obstetricians tell patients to go try again."[1] Because of this, many couples with secondary infertility never see a specialist. It has been reported that only two out of five couples with secondary infertility (40 percent), compared with two out of three couples with primary infertility (66 percent), ever receive medical treatment.[2]

Those with recurring infertility are more apt to seek treatment. Nonetheless, many respondents tell of doctors who relied on whatever treatment had worked in the past and who "kept handing out Clomid" or performed thirteen IUIs before reexamining the problem. For others, however, the knowledge gained through prior infertility is a definite asset the second time around:

> This time, we didn't waste time, and I felt totally in control. I told my doctor what I felt I needed, and fortunately he went along with me each step. . . . I felt more in control, knowing what to expect in treatment.

Note: It is important to point out that in this case, the patient was dealing with recurring endometriosis (the presence of endometrial tissue in other than normal locations, e.g., the ovaries or fallopian tubes) and sought treatment as soon as she wanted to conceive.

Minimizing the Problem

Diane Clapp sees more denial of and resistance to the diagnosis among those with secondary infertility than among their childless counterparts: "They often don't realize that fertility changes. There is a lot of disbelief, and the assumption is that 'I've done it once, I can do it again.' "³ This thought is certainly logical; unfortunately, as you know, such logic is based on a faulty premise.

Data indicate a higher pregnancy rate among those with secondary as opposed to primary infertility. A study of possible predictors of infertility outcomes found that a prior pregnancy with the same partner was the "single most powerful positive factor associated with pregnancy."⁴ Yet each case is different, and a higher statistical success rate is no rationale for a wait-and-see approach. It is difficult to overcome your own natural reluctance and denial in order to push for the necessary diagnostic testing and treatment; however, many patients report that they, rather than their doctors, provided the impetus to go forward. Some doctors resist such input and feel that their patients are overreacting: One woman describes her doctor as "impatient and irritated" at her feelings of discouragement, which he felt were unjustified and premature.

While some doctors are said to be well aware of secondary infertility and advise their patients of the possibility, others do not take the problem seriously, providing reassurances and advice to relax and not worry. Besides failing to validate your concerns, such misplaced confidence can result in lost time and raised expectations. The following account describes one such scenario:

> Looking back, it frustrates me that at first doctors didn't take the problem seriously when I was worried after not conceiving after six months or when I reported again after a year of trying. They just said, "You've gotten pregnant before." They either didn't have any concept how common a problem secondary infertility is OR chose not to inform me. Their attitude kept me from taking the problem as seriously as I could have, and as a result, advice of "Just go home and relax for a year" was taken and years were wasted because of it.

Similarly, another woman with a problem that would make pregnancy extremely unlikely without intervention did not learn this until after years of trying to conceive:

> [Each year at the annual exam,] I was told, "Your timing must be off," "You are trying too hard," "Your husband is working nights during your fertile time," etc., etc., etc., ad nauseam. Finally, after three years

of being told excuses, I insisted something was wrong with me, and had a
. . . laparoscopy. I had total blockage of my left tube, partial of my right.

In other cases, false reassurances can cause additional losses that
might have been prevented or even a worsening of the problem. A
woman who described her doctor's approach as "not aggressive"
later learned that she had endometriosis, a condition that worsens
with time. Another woman who had experienced two miscarriages
was told, "This is very 'normal'; don't worry; everything is *probably* fine." After her third miscarriage, she was again told, "You have
excellent chances of having a baby next time—just try again." Trying again can sometimes carry more emotional than medical risks.

Diagnosing the Problem

If your doctor feels that there may not be a medical problem, and
that conception will occur, she or he might be reluctant to subject
you to invasive and expensive testing. On the other hand, if you are
already concerned about your fertility and have a gut feeling that
something is wrong, you may wonder why your case does not war-
rant more attention:

> We were very surprised by the work-up. Since we were dealing with
> secondary infertility, no physical examinations were performed; just a
> detailed history was taken. Then, some days later, blood was drawn for
> a progesterone and prolactin level. When this was normal, my husband
> spoke to the doctor and got the advice "Keep trying." After all my
> reading and thinking about infertility, I found this amazing.

In other cases, mistaken understanding of certain conditions may
cause them to be ruled out as potential problems. For instance, endometriosis is commonly considered a "career woman's disease"
that is prevented by pregnancy and frequently seen in older women
trying to have children. Another view, however, is that "delayed
childbearing has no bearing on whether or not a woman will develop endometriosis. . . . [P]eople who had babies when they were
young [can] get endometriosis in their thirties." Similarly, a doctor
continues: "Most of my patients who are diagnosed with endometriosis have already been pregnant and delivered babies. . . .
So it is basically a disease of fertile women, not infertile women. . . .

Pregnancy doesn't provide any protection at all."[5] Medical articles that perpetuate the attitude that "pregnancy tends to prevent the development of endometriosis"[6] could lead doctors to overlook this diagnosis for patients with secondary infertility, as seen in the following account:

> I don't feel that the medical field has served me particularly well, especially since it's taken four-and-a-half years to diagnose endometriosis. . . . I have also felt that they are good doctors—but the treatment of infertility is no more than highly educated guesswork.

(It is unclear in this case whether the speaker is referring to an OB/GYN with a general practice or to an infertility specialist. But even the latter would probably acknowledge that while more and more is known about infertility, much remains to be learned.) An article in the RESOLVE national newsletter highlights the confusion about possible causes of secondary infertility: "Certainly some problems, such as congenital absence of the vas deferens, anovulation and endometriosis are *unlikely* in couples with previous conceptions; however, a previous pregnancy does not *rule out* a male factor, ovulatory dysfunction or endometriosis. [Emphasis added]."[7]

Among respondents for this book, male factors were the most commonly reported cause of the infertility, followed by unexplained infertility. While this finding is not representative, it points to the need for a careful and thorough evaluation of both partners. The lack of a diagnosis raises special issues for doctors and patients. One woman with unexplained infertility describes the impact of not having a concrete diagnosis:

> After talking to many women with secondary infertility, it seems that . . . many of us have been placed in the "unexplained infertility" group. . . . This too makes the infertility more baffling for me, as I keep wondering if maybe at some level I may be "causing" my infertility because of the stress of working outside the home, raising a small child, and trying too hard to conceive. It might be easier if the reason could be pinpointed.

After her second miscarriage, another woman searches for a reason,

> Everyone, it seemed, needed an explanation—a reason WHY it happened, or they had a reason for us—"You shouldn't have been lifting

and holding your son," "You shouldn't have been painting." . . . These words only compounded the sorrow and the searching in myself of WHY? It HAS to be something that I have done or not done properly for this to happen to us again.

In cases of unexplained infertility, it would be helpful if doctors explained that while current technology may be unable to pinpoint the problem, that does not mean a medical problem doesn't exist. Receiving a diagnosis and possible treatment options enables couples to get on with their lives as illustrated below:

> We learned . . . that my remaining tube was basically useless and that my chances of natural pregnancy were zero, short of a miracle. In vitro fertilization or adoption was our only chance. We checked in vitro out and could not afford the cost or the emotional upheaval.

This couple was able to adopt soon after they contacted a lawyer.

The lack of a thorough evaluation of both partners can result in needlessly wasted time, money, energy, and hope. One woman relates with chagrin how a male factor was identified after two years:

> I had such mixed emotions. Now I know the reason for the problems. . . . If this information was secured a year ago, the five Pergonal cycles, hysteroscopy, and definitely the GIFT would never have been done.

In some cases, the lack of insurance coverage limits the infertility work-up and your options for treatment. The expense of infertility treatments has becomes a dominant theme in medical decision making, enabling some couples to pursue treatment, while others with the same prognosis cannot:

> A specialist said IVF was our only hope. It was not even *touched* by insurance in Ohio. But I felt so sure—because we were otherwise so *healthy* and young—IVF would work for us. So we paid almost $6,000 for an IVF cycle.

> Up until I was about forty, I seriously considered all of the newest alternative means, such as donated embryo, surrogate mother, donating *my* embryo to be carried by another woman, etc. But these options are all $20,000± and we do not have that kind of money. . . . If [infertility] was covered, even partially, I know I would have continued IVF treatments until I realized my dream of giving birth to my second child. To deny women this coverage is unconscionable.

The lack of payment for technology that could lead to the birth of a child stirs deep resentment and anger and may be viewed as "unconscionable" when considered in light of the fact that maternity benefits, abortion, and even sterilization are covered. Those struggling to conceive do not consider this "elective" and are angered by comparisons of infertility treatment to hair transplants, plastic surgery, or sex-change operations. Hopefully, national health insurance will have addressed these inequities.

Evaluating Your Treatment Experience

It may be difficult for you to evaluate the effectiveness of the medical care you are receiving; however, you are the only experts when it comes to how you are reacting to the treatment. Some patients have the cynical perspective that doctors do not care about how the treatments are affecting them so long as they keep coming back:

> The most underdeveloped aspect of infertility treatment is the psychological toll it exacts from the patient. Who is studying that? Certainly, it is in the best interest of reproductive endocrinologists to steer clear of the emotional price patients pay. . . . The bad news might be a deterrent to treatment for some. Better to lead naive patients down the unwieldy path of needles, sonograms, hope, and failure without a clear idea of how much it can hurt.

Still, many are concerned about the emotional costs to patients and advise couples to discontinue treatment if it is affecting them adversely:

> The quality of time you spend in infertility treatment is more important than the quantity of time. You must be able to honestly evaluate if you are benefiting from these energies or suffering from them. . . . Some couples continue with infertility treatment to the detriment of all other aspects of life; they have invested so much time and energy that to stop feels like total defeat. . . . Taking this step may actually signal that you have been successful and comfortable with your own limitations and priorities. You have recognized the need to go on with other aspects of your life and you have rewarded yourself with taking action to meet that end. This does not mean to say that you are not sad, angry, or disappointed, but you are not a failure if you have not achieved a pregnancy after one, five, or twenty years of trying.[8]

Need for a Specialist

While you may delay leaving your obstetrician because of both your personal relationship with him or her and your reluctance to enter the world of infertility treatment, many patients feel that OB/GYNs do not have all the technical expertise necessary. Diane Clapp explains that Reproductive endocrinology is a board sub-specialty of OB/GYN, which requires two years of training, and oral and written boards. She adds that infertility specialists rarely have a practice which includes obstetrics.

Some patients complain that it wasn't until they saw a specialist that they realized their previous doctors did not know how to time an endometrial biopsy or take prolactin levels. It is discouraging to have a laparoscopy performed by your doctor, only to need to have the surgery repeated by a specialist. Similarly, women have wasted years taking fertility drugs, only to learn later that they could not have conceived due to another, previously undiagnosed problem. One patient advises others:

> I recommend a specialist to anyone with the problem, primary or secondary. I think that OBs frankly don't know enough, aren't equipped for weekend ovulation, etc. And I think it is difficult to sit in a waiting room with a pregnant woman. . . . At any rate, it wasn't until our third doctor that we were given some diagnosis for the first time.
>
> I think I have learned a lot about being a consumer, especially a medical consumer, and I am less likely to stay with a physician if I don't like him or her. . . . I see this as a good outcome of being an infertility patient.

Doctors aren't all-knowing or infallible; most try to do their best for their patients, given their level of expertise and the current state of knowledge. Diagnosis and treatment do entail a certain degree of trial and error. No one doctor has all the answers to every case. It is important for you to be informed and to seek second opinions with specialists for an additional perspective on your care. (Lists of doctors specializing in infertility are available from RESOLVE, Inc., and the American Fertility Society.)

The Doctor-Patient Relationship

Isaac Schiff, M.D., is chief of gynecology and obstetrics at Massachusetts General Hospital in Boston. In the foreword to Menning's *Infertility: A Guide for the Childless Couple*, Schiff, as a physician experienced in treating infertility patients, writes:

> It is a wise infertility specialist who realizes that one can only give so much education and emotional support in the course of daily care. We would like to give more, and we are often frustrated because we cannot. Those of us who have referred patients to RESOLVE support groups have benefited from their educated approach to their case, their desire to be full participants, and their demands to be respectfully and carefully managed. . . . I am aware in the beginning there are often "war stories" about anger at their physicians' handling of the case, miscommunications, and lack of emotional support. But RESOLVE groups are not formed just to encourage anger and catharsis, but to hold each individual and couple responsible for asking for what they need and for trying to achieve it. . . . These couples become better patients by educating themselves and being encouraged to suggest helpful changes in their care. The days of "doctor as God" are over. Doctor as "partner in care" has come of age. We ought to be very grateful.[9]

While we may applaud Dr. Schiff's perspective, the era of doctor as "partner in care" in many cases has yet to be realized. There are many imbalances in the doctor-patient relationship. Although doctors may no longer be viewed as omnipotent gods, usually they possess superior education, information, and training; patients are at a real disadvantage in keeping up with a highly technical and changing field. Some patients, particularly those with a limited education, are awed by the perceived gap in status between themselves and their physician. Many feel overwhelmed at the prospect of learning what appears to be a new language of treatment and entering unknown and uncharted territory. Finally, in many cases there remains a gender gap between male physicians and predominantly female patients, a factor that can add to the power imbalance and differing perspectives.

An inevitable but crucial difference between you and your medical providers is your personal investment in the outcome. You view both procedures and their results differently from your doctor. Doctors perform procedures repeatedly; they are trained to be objective and matter-of-fact. Some may underestimate the discomfort caused by a certain procedure or see an insemination as routine while you see it as the possible moment of conception. Similarly, a miscarriage is not just a "statistical aberration" but the loss of your future child. When you have so much invested in the results of your treatment, you can become frustrated with your doctors' comparative indifference—you are literally fighting for your longed-for child and to regain control of your lives.

Many doctors do care a great deal about their patients' well-being, even sharing their pain and frustration. They want to succeed in helping their patients conceive, and some experience their inability to do so as a personal failure. At times, they too may feel discouraged and not in control when treatments do not work out as they had hoped. Even so, it is neither realistic nor desirable for doctors to experience the same degree of emotional devastation as their patients. Doctors may treat dozens of infertile couples a day—all of whom are under stress and looking to the physician for a solution. The cumulative effect of sharing in so much emotion would be overwhelming. To remain effective, doctors need to focus on the treatment they can provide and realize that "success" may lie in providing the best possible care, not just in achieving a successful pregnancy.

Other dynamics can complicate the doctor-patient relationship. You may resent being dependent on a doctor to achieve what you may earlier have achieved on your own. In addition, out of necessity, the doctor becomes a party to your sexual lives and compromises your privacy: "I was (and am) a private person. I could talk about my body, but didn't [feel comfortable] recording details of when my husband and I were intimate, knowing that someone else would be looking at it." Husbands sometimes feel jealousy toward the physician, who may be seen as usurping their role of getting their wives pregnant.

You may find yourself using magical thinking, leading you to believe that somehow your doctor actually knows whether or not you will become pregnant. This makes you particularly vulnerable to your doctor's opinions and gives the doctor's words, intonations, and even facial expressions tremendous weight. When doctors are being encouraging, most patients want to believe they are right:

[My doctor] all but promised us a pregnancy. In fact, he went so far as to say he had never had a case of secondary infertility that had not resulted in a pregnancy.

Although the words were certainly meant kindly, clearly this woman and her spouse were less prepared to face the reality of not becoming pregnant.

The anger characterizing infertility is in some cases inappropriately directed toward the caregivers, who are vulnerable as messengers of bad news. A patient describes her experience with IVF and blames the physician for what she perceived to be the false hope she was given. It is possible that, given her status of secondary infertility, she was told that she was a good candidate for IVF; it is easy for patients to misinterpret encouragement as a guarantee:

It was a nightmare! Not physically, I could bear that, but mentally it was the worst crisis I faced so far. . . . I blamed the IVF doctor because he gave me hope, then it was crashed into nothing.

You may find, regardless of your level of sophistication or cynicism, that on some level you crave a special relationship with your medical providers. The medical team may be the only people who know that you are experiencing infertility. You may look to the doctor not only for a medical diagnosis but also to validate your reactions and to reassure you that you are not "crazy" and are handling the situation adequately. It would be very reassuring to many if medical providers raised issues that might be worrisome but difficult to express, such as sexual functioning, strain in the relationship, and the emotional side effects of medications.

Building a Relationship with Your Providers

As a patient, you may feel vulnerable, needy, and dependent on the doctor's expertise. (Doctors themselves who become patients are especially cognizant of these feelings.) Investing the doctor with so much power over your life goals is a burden for everyone. As Dr. Schiff suggests, the role of savior or seer is a heavy one for doctors to carry. One way to avoid this trap is for you to educate and empower yourself. Doctors can help by providing resources and referrals and by encouraging such a collaborative approach.

When you consider working with a medical team, it is helpful to learn what their groundrules and procedures are: Is there a call-in hour? Are calls routinely handled by a nurse? What is the staffing coverage for IUIs? Will your own doctor be performing procedures, or is there a team? What insurance do they accept? Do they have a staff member who handles claims? What is the wait for an appointment? What is their policy about children in the waiting rooms? Is there a staff member who can watch your child during a procedure?

When you meet with the doctor—and sometimes couples meet with a few before they decide—do you get a sense that your styles mesh? How comfortable is the doctor with patient input? Can you anticipate any potential conflicts? What are your expectations of the doctor, and are they realistic? How accessible will the doctor be, and in what situations? What trade-offs can you handle, if necessary, between technical expertise and personal attention? What is most important to you and to your partner?

Once you begin treatment, it is important to schedule periodic "taking stock" consultations with both of you and the doctor to do some joint planning and perhaps establish a flexible timeline for treatment. While such timelines are frequently amended, it is helpful to know that there is an endpoint. It is important to remember that you can control the pacing and that it is all right to take a break from treatment.

It is impossible for doctors to address fears that remain unarticulated, but sometimes patients lack the words to voice their unfocused concerns or fear being a bother. If you educate yourself and are aware of what to watch for, you can express your concerns and even aid in the diagnosis by picking up on subtle cues. Often a person knows something is wrong before hearing confirming test results. Many patients lack knowledge of what could be happening to their bodies. A study of women with early cessation of ovarian function (better known as premature ovarian failure or early menopause), 50 percent of whom were mothers, found that none knew that such a problem was possible.[10]

Some women are embarrassed that they know so little about fertility:

With secondary infertility, I find that doctors tend to expect a level of knowledge of the subject that I frankly don't have, not having undergone treatment for primary infertility. I feel silly asking simple questions about timing and hormones, but doctors really can't assume that you know all this stuff just because you've gotten pregnant.

In fact, those who have had trouble getting pregnant are more apt to have such a technical understanding of reproduction than those for whom the pregnancy "just happened."

It is important to overcome your embarrassment and ask questions until all of the information you are given or ask for is understandable. Often what the doctor says is not what you hear. Even couples who attend a consultation together frequently come away with differing assessments of the meaning of what has been said. This communication gap between professionals and patients is epitomized by a poignant misunderstanding in which a woman, having been told that her pregnancy was ectopic and that the tube had been removed, then asked if her baby was all right.

As patients, it is vital that you find out about the risks and side effects of any medications that you take. Some doctors are reluctant to suggest what might never occur; the problem is that if symptoms do arise, you might fail to associate them with the medications and worry needlessly that something is wrong with you. If you do feel side effects from the medications, including emotional reactions, you should inform your doctor. Sometimes patients are reluctant to do this, wishing to continue treatment at all costs; however, a change of dosage or medication might be all that's necessary.

One common difficulty is trying to make informed decisions based on what you feel are incomplete data. "But what is the likelihood of success for *us*?" is a familiar refrain. Doctors often feel frustrated when they cannot answer a specific question with any degree of certainty. As patients, you might welcome your doctors' admission of the limits of their knowledge and prefer realism to any false reassurances.

As a patient, you might appreciate a doctor who suggests getting another opinion, or refers you elsewhere for a specialized intervention. Usually, however, the burden for suggesting another opinion falls on patients, who often feel awkward or guilty about "abandoning" their physicians or questioning their advice. Getting another opinion is your right, and you need not feel apologetic or believe you are showing a lack of trust in your doctor if you pursue that option. A fresh perspective is beneficial regardless of the expertise of your physician, and such a step should not be seen as reflecting negatively on your treatment to date.

It can be empowering when you are told that there is no one right or wrong way to proceed, but rather instructed to use the available data to weigh the pros and cons and decide what is right for you and your family; however, the lack of clear-cut guidelines and the common disagreements about treatment, even among specialists, can be confusing and overwhelming. How can you be expected to decide when even the experts don't agree? Some couples prefer that their doctors take charge and feel that they are not up to taking on such a responsibility. When you are in crisis, it can be comforting to be told what to do. Yet while doctors do have the technical expertise, they cannot know without your input what pacing of the tests and procedures feels most comfortable, what degree of intervention you can handle and for how long, how you and your partner are coping with the infertility, what affect the medications have on you, and what your goals are as a family. Everyone evaluates treatment decisions differently. When a woman discontinues Pergonal because she feels its side effects make her unable to be a good mother, we see that treatment decisions involve more than statistical success rates. Similarly, while donor ovum or donor sperm may be the next step medically, these are issues of a very personal nature for a family to work through, usually with the assistance of professional counseling.

It is important that you try to give your doctor a sense of who you are outside of your diagnosis and how the infertility is affecting other aspects of your life. While doctors cannot be expected to meet your emotional as well as medical needs, they can be sensitive to the emotional dynamics of the situation and should be aware of other stresses in your life. Some doctors, realizing the strain of an infertility investigation, have staff members who provide counseling and/or refer patients routinely to RESOLVE support groups or therapists specializing in infertility. Others may be reluctant to refer patients automatically for supportive counseling, fearing that patients may feel stigmatized. Asking a doctor for a referral for emotional support is perfectly appropriate, however; most have local resources available.

A critical decision you may make with your doctor is at what point to discontinue treatment. Find out ahead of time what the success rate for each treatment is for your diagnosis and in your age-group, and whether the success rate goes down after a certain number of trials. It is important that you feel you have given treatment a fair trial; however, given today's technology, treatment options may never be exhausted. You must realistically weigh the costs—emotional, financial, and physical—against the likelihood of a successful pregnancy. (This dilemma is discussed more fully in Chapter 9, "Considering Possible Outcomes.") Discontinuing treatment can be hard particularly if you have developed relationships within the practice. Some patients report missing the support and attention which accompany treatment. Others do not want to disappoint the doctor and staff by "dropping out." Being able to discuss your situation frankly with your doctor and with all concerned is vital. No one treatment course is right for everyone, so while your doctor may be enthusiastic, ultimately you must decide whether or not a particular treatment makes sense for you.

The success of the doctor-patient relationship depends not only on achieving a pregnancy but also on the quality of the interaction. If, as patients, you take the responsibility for being informed and for making your needs known, and if you feel that you in turn have been treated with respect and received the best possible care, you are more apt to emerge from the infertility process feeling good about yourselves, whether or not you have a successful pregnancy.

9

Considering Possible Outcomes

The alternative to defining your life according to what you don't have—is to define your life according to what you do have and can have.

—Jean and Michael Carter
Sweet Grapes: How to Stop Being Infertile and Start Living Again

Often when you are pursuing a goal, it is impossible to focus on the benefits of other outcomes. For some, the very fact that the goal eludes them makes it even more cherished as an ideal. Somehow, considering the positives seems to be admitting defeat. Few outcomes are all positive or all negative, however, although it is hard to step back and see this when you are intent on achieving a deeply held goal. Sometimes it takes a chance to grieve for what may not occur before you can acknowledge the benefits of other options.

Couples experiencing primary infertility have a difficult time weighing their options; usually, however, they are clear about what their options are: treatment, adoption, third-party reproductive alternatives, or life without parenting. Certainly, the last alternative does not exist for couples who already have children. The other alternatives are also confounded because of the existing child or children: There are more people and dynamics to consider in the decision-making process. Ideas about the spacing of siblings sometimes may increase the sense of urgency in reaching a decision. Financial considerations are a real factor in both treatment and adoption decisions. As parents experiencing infertility you do, however, have one choice not available to childless infertile couples: You can make a conscious decision to parent your family the way it is.

You and your partner may be inclined to weigh the alternatives differently at different points in time; what is important is that you

133

reach a decision that works for your own family. There is no one correct outcome or way to feel about these possibilities. Family building is a personal and individual matter; you will reach different decisions based on your own backgrounds, resources, and feelings about families in general and your own family in particular.

Treatment Issues

Today when so many treatment options are available, it is hard to know whether or not to enter treatment and, if you do, when to put an end to it. You may feel torn between your desire for another successful pregnancy and another child and your feelings of responsibility to your existing child. It is hard to divide your resources, both emotional and financial, between the child you have and the child you long for. Some parents decide to stop treatment because they feel they need to be more accessible to their child; others, because they feel they cannot justify the expense.

The following story of a woman who pursued treatment for primary infertility but not for secondary infertility describes how her work/parenting choice limited her options the second time around:

> We always wanted a large family, so we started right away trying to get pregnant. . . . After many, many tests—to a tune of about $20,000—and surgery, I finally became pregnant . . . and went on to deliver a healthy baby girl. . . . She was pure *joy* in our lives. . . . We've never had any more children, though we have tried and tried on our own. I never did go back to the infertility specialist again, mainly because I quit work to stay home and be a full-time mother to this baby I had so desperately wanted. . . . So therefore our income was not at the level it was with two of us working. Due to the financial strain in seeing an infertility specialist, I did not go back for treatment of secondary infertility.

Another woman states that financial reasons were the determining factor in stopping treatment and instead pursuing adoption:

> Eventually we reached a point in our treatment where we were urged to try the Pergonal drug at a cost of $1,000 per month. We were also told that I would be an excellent candidate for ovum donation. We were very interested in this also. We did not have insurance coverage for any infertility treatment, and this factor colored our decision more

than anything to stop treatment. It was also becoming increasingly difficult to travel to the doctor's office every month. Arranging for childcare and traveling time shot the whole day. . . . The bottom line on our decision to give up treatment was a financial one. Had we had unlimited funds, we would have continued trying some of the high-tech procedures, and even now, almost four years later, wonder if we should have tried. . . . At this time, my husband and I are pursuing adoption. . . . It is a happy prospect.

Yet the decision is often not solely financial, as alluded to above and more explicitly in these words: "I am working with a gynecologist, not an infertility expert. Although I don't really feel that I am getting the best care that way, it's hard for me to take the time, energy, and money needed to go to experts." Another woman who is experiencing recurring infertility describes the specific daily hardships in combining treatment and parenting, such as being unable to rest after receiving her Pergonal injection, hearing her son crying for her in the morning while she needs to remain still and take her temperature, and relying on her husband more to take care of their son. These are problems she didn't have the first time she was in treatment. Some women find that the angry outbursts triggered by their reaction to hormones affect their relationship with their children. Some discontinue treatment, stating that they "couldn't parent well with these negative emotions." (See Chapter 7, "Other Parenting Concerns.")

For some, the determination to stop treatment and pursue other options such as adoption comes more easily, particularly if assisted reproductive technology is not being considered:

I conceived our son the *first month* my husband and I tried (with great surprise). . . . Our son is now six-and-a-half years old. We started trying for a second when he was two (assuming we would have no trouble). . . . Almost five years have gone by now. . . . We began infertility testing after one year of trying, and since then have received a variety of reasons for our infertility. . . . About a year ago, we pursued IUI with Clomid for three cycles and gave up and made our decision to pursue an international adoption (Korea) last fall. We had already decided not to pursue high-tech treatments like IVF. . . . Right now, we are hoping that our adoption will come through.

Other parents feel they absolutely must conceive another child, by whatever means. One woman who was in a quandary about whether or not to pursue treatment relates a dream she had about the dilemma: "I see two elderly ladies on a sunny park bench and spill the story to them. One of the ladies stops me midway and simply says, 'You'll never be sorry you had another baby.'" She goes on to recount her belief that the ladies are symbols of wisdom who have lived their lives and can look back and make valuable judgments. Deciding to take their advice and describing an additional family member as the greatest "investment" they could make, she is pursuing IVF and "backing up my options with donor eggs, and lastly a surrogate."

Couples who do pursue advanced reproductive technology often liken it to a rollercoaster and frequently find it hard to make the decision to end treatment and move on to other alternatives. The following excerpts, taken from a journal kept by a woman throughout her infertility treatment, illustrate why it is not easy for many to stop treatment or "just adopt," as others may suggest. This saga is long, but so is the journey undertaken by so many couples. The very complexity of this one account parallels the ups and downs of treatment that complicate the decision-making process for many couples.

August 1991

It took three years to get to this point [IVF]. So many ups and downs, tears of happiness, fear, and despair. I became involved in two different RESOLVE support groups to deal with the many emotions aroused by infertility.... I spoke frequently about adoption and contacted the Polish consulate to get information.... In essence, the last three years have been all consumed by tests, procedures, medications, and prayers to add to our family.

When I finally became pregnant, I lost my longed-for baby at seven weeks. I was pregnant for Christmas and without child by New Year's.... I lost another pregnancy ... days after my thirty-eighth birthday. Now I worried that I would never have a pregnancy come to term. But I couldn't get off the merry-go-round, even though adoption became increasingly appealing to me.

I wanted to hold to what I was saying all along: that the GIFT would be my last attempt at fertility. But I had traveled that long, painful road for so long, I just couldn't call it quits.... I knew IVF was my next step.

So onto the rollercoaster I go, . . . faster and more daring than the merry-go-round I have been on for two years. I hope I know when to get off this time, . . . for now I am thirty-nine years old and very tired and burned-out.

September 1991
I got my period on the tenth day after the transfer. . . . I felt a black shade being pulled down—this is the end: of fertility treatments, . . . of any hope of having a biological child. . . . I was so despondent that I had to just park on the road and sob.

I find myself crying again in the car while driving to the fertility clinic. I prepare my "goodbye" speech to the doctor and his staff in between the tears. "Thank you for all your support, . . . but I have had it! No more intervention!"

However, my doctor's reaction was that I had had a "chemical pregnancy" which could not last and "to look at it as being a positive sign, . . . encouraging; . . . chances are better next time it may be a good pregnancy." So instead of saying goodbye, I found myself planning my next IVF cycle. . . . I was in tears when I left—what a horrible tease! When I was just ready to give up, I find myself jumping back on the merry-go-round.

[Surprisingly, pregnancy tests continued to get stronger—"just where supposed to be."]

Well, bounce those emotions again! . . . I was pregnant! So the next two weeks became increasingly more stressful. The hormone count was slowly creeping up rather than doubling. . . . I was living for the next lab value; . . . the conversations with the embryologist . . . leaned toward the possibility of a blighted ovum. . . .

I begged for a sonogram. . . . The suspense was keeping me up at night . . . and was making me miserable to be around in the day. And the major, major miracle was that little heartbeat! . . .

So . . . one day at a time. Stress has my eczema full-blown. . . . So I continue scratching, praying, and hoping that someday I'll admire the near-perfect angel that I have wanted for so long, worked so hard for, gave up hopes for, and now am an emotional mess about. But it will all be worth it in the end. . . . I just hope this is not just a tease.

A Week Later—September 1991
Yes, it was a horrible tease, . . . so close, yet today all my fears and anxieties came to an end.

At exactly seven weeks after the transfer, I went for another sonogram. . . . The conclusion was that there was no heartbeat. . . . I was
again living my worst fears—another lost pregnancy.

It seems this should mark the end. Enough is enough!

July 1993
However, this was not the end of the story. I went for another IVF
cycle [and later implantation of frozen embryos]. I painfully made the
decision to stop any further intervention. . . . I still carry the unfulfilled
dream of again becoming pregnant. I am now forty-one years old and
realize that another pregnancy is near impossible. . . .

However, we probably will be traveling to Poland to adopt . . . and
very possibly will be closing this chapter to our life: the long, painful,
and tormenting five years of wanting to complete our family. I sincere-
ly hope that we will be ending this story with the adorable blond-
haired, blue-eyed little girl we have in our photos.

The fact that in this case there was continual reason to hope served
to delay the decision to adopt. You may find yourself in this position, with technology offering you yet another treatment to try.
Making the decision to stop treatment is difficult when a successful
pregnancy might be just one more cycle away. Not deciding, however, carries the risk of remaining in limbo and drifting rather than
actively choosing an alternative. Specific issues about treatment are
discussed in both *Beyond Infertility: The New Paths to Parenthood*
by Susan Cooper and Ellen Glazer and in *Taking Charge of Infertility* by Pat Johnston.

Issues in Considering Adopting

Adoption in some ways may resemble the rollercoaster of treatment, but with one crucial exception: Despite the uncertainty,
those who pursue adoption steadfastly and flexibly almost always
have a success rate of 100 percent. One bioadoptive mother recalls
how she felt before and during the adoption process:

Adoption was not something that excited me at first. It seemed to be a
simple answer for others to give me. . . . And yet I knew that we wanted more children. . . .

Adoption became something I dealt with on two levels, one business, the other emotional. It can sound very cruel talking about fees and services . . . but it needs to be done. On the emotional side, there were many times that I would cry for our loss, the pain of the birthfamily, the separation for the child, and also just having a chance to parent another child.

It took some thought filling out questions on background, personality, and family life. The process would be good for all prospective parents. In some ways, it might have been easier for us to fill out because we knew what we were like as parents, and that took some pressure off. Still, it was somewhat different from our first path to parenthood.

It was while we were awaiting the adoption that people seemed most comfortable talking with us about our search for another child. The impression I got was that it was easier to speak of adoption with its upcoming joy than [of] the pain associated with infertility.

Our phone call came when we least expected it, in the middle of Labor Day weekend, just after we had torn apart the kitchen to strip and refinish the cabinets. Fortunately, we had been given three days' notice [instead of twenty-four hours], as travel to another state was involved.

Adoption is a complex decision for any couple to make. There are many types of adoptions to consider, such as; traditional, open, international, parent initiated and special needs. For most people, adoption is not a first choice since they have grown up assuming they would reproduce. Often much grieving and soul-searching occur before people realize that it is a workable option for them. Some couples only consider adoption after they have exhausted medical possibilities; others prefer to pursue adoption and treatment simultaneously or alternate between the two. Treatment and adoption can both be draining; however, some couples reason that the more avenues they try, the sooner they will succeed.

It is important to understand what your motivations are for wanting another child: whether it is to parent another child, to experience pregnancy and childbirth again, or to produce another child together. Some needs are more readily met through adoption. This section will include varying perspectives on adoption from women throughout the decision-making continuum. Some of these women have adopted or will go on to adopt; some are just beginning to consider the possibility; others may decide against buiding their families through adoption. Their feelings about adoption are heartfelt often reflecting their ambivalence and sometimes anger and grief. It is important to remember that adoption decision-making is a process and feelings change over time.

A difference exists between adoption as the only route to parenthood and adoption as a way of increasing family size. While the vast majority of women say they would consider adopting if they were childless,[1] the decision is less automatic for those who already have a child. One woman airs her fears about adoption, "I am a mother; I am mothering every day. I don't have to take the risks of adoption since I am already a mother. . . . I worry about getting a child [who] is disruptive [and] who makes my child's life uncomfortable." Acknowledging negative fantasies about adoption is the only way to place them in perspective. This woman is still considering adoption as an option, but realizes she is not yet ready to pursue it.

Theoretically, parents might be expected to be more open to adding to their families through adoption for two reasons: First, they know the satisfactions of raising children and are confident of their ability to parent and, second, having once reproduced, they might be better able to focus on the parenting as opposed to the genetic continuity motivations for having children. Pat Johnston emphasizes that the desire to parent is the key to successful adoption and that the child must be accepted for who he or she is, not as a substitute for the child a couple wished to have.

Some mothers are clear that they want to parent another child and are eager to pursue adoption. One woman in the middle of an IVF cycle said that she would not even return for the reimplantation of her embryos if her husband would agree to adopt. It seems that women are often ready to adopt before their husbands reach that point, perhaps due to a greater desire to parent another child or to the time lag discussed in Chapter 3.

One woman whose husband couldn't even discuss adoption persuaded him to join a RESOLVE support group, and in this way he became aware of her "deep desire to have another child and [her] despair from all [her] futile attempts." For many couples, discussions about adoption are a start-and-stop proposition, beginning with a reluctance to consider the option, advancing to a commitment to think about thinking about it, and progressing to actually considering adoption as a viable alternative. But few couples proceed through these stages in tandem. It is likely, that you will approach and retreat from the subject, depending on your optimism or pessimism each month and your respective commitment to having another child. While at times disagreements about the desirability of adopting may appear to be insoluble because both partners' positions are deeply held, some of even the most intractable impasses have been resolved through couples therapy.

Many people who feel they could easily parent just an adopted child have concerns about adopting after having given birth. Some find themselves at a disadvantage in the adoption process because they have a child. Still others have concerns about justifying the expense when the money could be used for their existing child's education. By the time they are seeking to adopt a second child, some couples experience difficulty because they are older:

> People ask me, "Why don't you adopt?" They cannot believe what I've gone through and make me feel like I'm dragging my whole family down by hanging on to [my] dream. I could explain that I talked to adoption groups four years ago and they told me then my husband and I were too old . . . and that we already had a child. . . . That left dealing with open adoption or adopting a handicapped child or a child of mixed [racial] background. People make me feel like I'm greedy for wanting a "perfect" child (meaning not handicapped) or that I'm closed-minded for not choosing to adopt a child of color into my home. These are usually the same people who have two or three children of their own. They did not have to rationalize their family planning.

Another couple, who had a fourteen-year-old biological child and had worked through their issues about adopting a child, felt stymied by adoption agency policies:

> I learned that because I had one biological child, Catholic Social Services would not even accept an adoption request from us, and most other "for profit" agencies told us we should be put behind those couples with *no* children. . . . If I could adopt a child—aged up to ten—I still am open to that. I still love children, and I do not feel, as I once did, that it has to be "mine" by means of conception, pregnancy, and giving birth.

Unfortunately, sometimes misinformation and/or fears about the difficulty of adopting and even about the home-study process discourage couples who have considered adoption from pursuing this option:

> We started thinking a little about adoption, something I had never seri-
> ously considered before. . . . I remember reading an article about adop-
> tion which described the couple as having to write book reports for
> their home study. So, whatever I've gone through since in pursing preg-
> nancy, I always say, "It's better than having to write book reports!"

For others, the infertility itself may be seen as a sign that they are
not meant to have another child, while their pain precludes being
open to alternatives:

> The thought of adopting someone else's child when I had to give up the
> dream of my own is too difficult. . . . When your ovaries are destroyed,
> does that mean you shouldn't have more? Should I never pursue adop-
> tion? Will the new baby be too much to handle?. . . .

Despite the obstacles, emotional or logistical, couples who do decide to adopt are almost always able to do so. Adoption has gotten
more flexible in recent years and there are now more resources
available. Although conventional wisdom may be to the contrary,
many birthmothers prefer to place their baby with a family in
which the child is assured of having siblings. Birthmothers too have
reservations about "only" children; however, most prospective
adopters fear that they will be at a disadvantage:

> Finally, when we tried to adopt, we felt also like "second-class citizens"
> because the fact that we had a biological child put us "lower on the list"
> or "less desirable" to birthparents.

The following account underscores that while adoption is for many
a wonderful form of family building, it is not a "cure" for infertility.[2]

> We did eventually adopt and have a beautiful family, but I will carry
> the pain of this experience with me forever. I have come to the conclu-
> sion that the only "resolution" or "resolve" regarding infertility is that I
> will carry this aching hole forever, that it is a piece of sorrow that is
> part of me (but hopefully not all of me) for the rest of my life.

The lingering ache does not mean that the child who was adopted
is less than accepted or that the parenting is less than satisfying; this
woman has honestly acknowledged the legacy infertility has left in
her life and is striving to put it into context. Similarly, for some giving birth following infertility does not erase the experience of hav-

ing been infertile. Many other women, however, find that adopting does take away the ache, particularly if they were motivated more by a desire to parent another child than by the wish to have another pregnancy, or give birth.

Becoming foster parents has met the parenting needs of some families,

> Zachary now has a foster brother and sister to fight with, although we do not know how long they will be staying with us. We went from one four-year-old to three kids—three, four, and five years old. What a change![3]

Concerns about Bonding

The attention paid to childbirth education today, while worthwhile, seems to overshadow the importance placed on parenting. Part of the rationale for natural childbirth is the increased emphasis placed on bonding. The term *attachment* conveys more of the sense of an ongoing parenting process than a single instance of bonding; attachments develop over time. A mother who has given birth and then adopted compares the experiences:

> Some mothers speak of instant bonding and love with their children. While I knew that I loved my first daughter, loving her for who she was didn't take place instantly. This time, I didn't have a clue what she would look like, and I would be just as strange to her as any other person. And yet I knew in time we would belong together.
>
> Our family fit has gone well. All four of us can't imagine what it would be like to not be together. There is no difference in the amount of love given to each child. The girls are very close as sisters, much closer than I had anticipated. . . . It would have been wonderful if I had had the privilege of being pregnant with my younger daughter, but that wouldn't cause me to love her any more than I do.

Parents often wonder whether they can attach to a later child as they have to their first. This is a concern whether the first child arrived by birth or adoption. Parents by both birth and adoption question whether or not they will be able to love a subsequent child as much as their first. Parents experiencing secondary infertility often attribute this fear of feeling differently about a subsequent child to the fact that their children might come into the family through different routes.

My husband might have agreed with my wish to adopt if we couldn't have any children, but it is a very hard decision for him now because he feels it would be unfair to an adopted child with our own boy as a standard. . . . After he has loved our boy wildly, he's afraid he couldn't love an adopted baby.

Parents usually feel differently about their children for one reason or other: birth order, gender or temperament. This does not mean that they aren't equally loved rather it enables each child to be treated as an individual.

If you are concerned about your ability to relate to a child whom you adopt, it is important to reality test this concern. Talking to other parents about their differing parenting experiences is one way to see whether or not this concern is normal ambivalence. One woman describes her concerns about attachment and the ways in which she dealt with them:

One of our biggest concerns was if we would be able to love another child as much as our daughter. It helped talking with friends who had adopted two children and then given birth, but we still could not be certain. It helped to also hear and read that this was a common question many parents had when preparing for a second child. We decided that as far as we could know it wouldn't be a problem, but we would have to wait for the reality of a child to really know.

The following research data places this concern into perspective.

Research on Bioadoptive Families

A survey of more than 1,000 mothers—biological, adoptive, and bioadoptive—compared adoptive and biological mothers and found virtually no difference in the quality of the mother-child relationships. Nor, as couples sometimes fear, did bioadoptive mothers feel closer to their biological child. About one-third of the adoptive mothers in this study had children by both birth and adoption; the mother-child relationships were just as close, just as strong, with the children who had been adopted as with the children born to them: "Not all wonderful relationships, but no better or worse than biological."[4] In fact, those women who also had given birth to children were reported to have "a psychological edge" over mothers who had only adopted children. With such firsthand experience of parenting both through adoption and birth, these women seemed to possess a feeling of security and confidence that they were as real a mother to the children whom they adopted as to the children to whom they had given birth.

The order in which the children would join prospective bio-adoptive families appears to be a significant factor in decision making. Clearly, the thought processes are different for a couple without children who adopt and then later become pregnant and give birth. (The reality that this popular myth does in fact occur is attributable to couples pursuing both adoption and treatment options and in no way implies that adoption itself somehow mystically causes a pregancy.) In order for you to decide to form a family with children you have both given birth to and adopted, you must confront concerns about your ability to parent equally, concerns that do not occur to parents who adopt their first child and do not anticipate later giving birth. On the other hand, a conscious decision to adopt following the birth of a child ideally sends a message to the child that she was wanted for herself not as a substitute for a biological child.

The Existing Child and the Adoption Process

Many parents face a quandary: They feel that their child is the best advertisement of their parenting abilities and would help them make their case to either agency workers or a birthmother; at the same time, they question the advisability of involving their child in the home-study process or, perhaps more problematic, in any meetings with a birthmother. Adoption policies vary. In cases of open adoption, wherein the parties are known to one another, such meetings are common. In other situations, parties may meet one another without sharing identifying information, whereas in traditional agency adoptions, the parties usually neither meet nor exchange identifying information. Yet, even in traditional confidential adoptions, birthmothers are increasingly encouraged to select adoptive parents based on a picturebook the latter prepare about themselves and on their written responses on the adoption application.

The uncertainty of adoption outcomes, particularly in cases of private or parent-initiated adoption, and the potentially long waiting period for a baby to arrive are both difficult for a child to cope with. One boy, whenever he was taken on errands with his mother, would ask if they were "going to pick up the baby." While adults also find it emotionally hard to accept the waiting and not knowing, cognitively, at least, they are better able to understand the process and the time sequence. Without a grasp of time and without the ability to distinguish wishes from reality, a child easily moves from "We're thinking about adopting a baby" to "A baby is coming to our house!" Children see their parents as all-powerful; after all, their parents are the ones they go to if they want something, and it's hard to imagine their parents can't have whatever they want. So once parents decide on adoption, children assume it will happen.

While the question of being chosen or approved of either by a birthparent or an agency is uncomfortable for many parents, it may raise different issues for a child. If the family is not chosen right away, the child may not understand and feel to blame. Still, a child is a vital part of the household and as such is part of the process. The best role for the child might well be a cameo supporting part: very low-key and in the background. For instance, the child could be introduced and then left to play while the adults talk. It might be advisable to have someone stay with the child to minimize interruptions. Some agency workers may not be used to conducting a home study in a family with a child; raising this issue ahead of time and brainstorming ways to involve the child might pave the way for the meeting.

Parents who are adopting should consider from the start what they plan to tell both the child they have and the one they are adopting about the adoption, about the reasons for it, and about the birthparents. The older sibling may play a role in telling the younger child the story of his or her arrival into the family; however, the details about their birthparents really belong to the children themselves. An increasingly common scenario is one in which the older child has met the birthparents and perhaps even birthsiblings, while the child being adopted might never have the opportunity to do so. Pat Johnston's *Adopting after Infertility* is a valuable resource in addressing adoption issues.

Parents may wonder about the impact of the concept of adoption on their children's feelings of permanence. If one woman cannot care for her child, might their own parents at some later date be unable to care for them? In explaining adoption to a child it is important to use appropriate adoption language. If the child realizes that an adoption plan is made by birthparents who are not ready to parent a child (or not able to parent another child), such fears should be alleviated, particularly if the parents point out that they have chosen to parent. What if a new baby has to be removed from the home before the adoption is finalized (every adoptive parent's worst nightmare)? Would a subsequent adopted sibling be viewed as less than a stable part of the family?

Some issues, while disquieting, can be prepared for and dealt with if the need arises. The best advice for parents is to be governed by their knowledge of their child; to be as honest and open as possible, timing and presenting information in an age-appropriate way that respects all parties in the adoption; and to avoid promising anything beyond their control. Children who have been a party to the adoption process may feel a special joy and sense of involvement if a new sibling joins their family.

Some parents feel that adopting an older child is a workable option for their families. The fact that they are already parents may give them the confidence to handle the challenges that often accompany the adoption of an older child. Depending on the age of their existing child, the adoption of an older child might best approximate their original hopes for the spacing of siblings. Pat Johnston advises parents considering this alternative to become well informed and well prepared by demanding all the information and supportive services available.

Issues in Third-Party Reproductive Options

Having conceived and given birth to at least one child together, you may be shocked if you learn that any future pregnancy must result from using a donor. This is a trying concept for anyone to grasp, particularly so when you have already produced one child together. Nevertheless, it is not uncommon for sperm counts to decrease or for a woman to experience early cessation of ovarian function or require a hysterectomy following an earlier pregnancy.

Deciding whether to try to achieve a pregnancy via collaborative reproduction such as donor sperm, donor ovum, or with a
surrogate raises issues common to both adoption and advanced
treatment and must also take into account the existing child. Couples must consider the investment of time and money in the procedures, as well as weigh their ability to accept a child who is biolog-
ically a half-sibling to their existing child. They must consider the
feelings of the nonbiologically related parent as well as questions
of privacy and openness vs. secrecy about the procedure. Some
couples attach great importance to equity, feeling it is crucial for
all parties to have the same biological relationship to one another.
Others feel that the genetic input and the chance to experience another pregnancy are overriding positives and that their parenting
will not be adversely affected by the different ways in which the
children were conceived. One woman describes her feelings about
pursuing donor insemination, as well as some of the issues raised
by that choice:

> Since [my husband's] decision to go with donor, I feel closer to him. I
> apreciate his ability to accept his infertility and to be a confident
> enough person to know he could love a child that is not genetically his,
> but is genetically mine. I know that he is doing this mainly out of his
> love for me and our family. . . .
>
> Right now, what I am struggling with is whether to go with frozen
> or fresh [sperm]. . . . I would ideally like to use fresh, with a donor
> who is willing to sign a release which would allow the child, when he
> or she is an adult, to obtain identifying information about him. But
> those two features together are not available to me.

Third party or collaborative reproductive techniques are best understood as an alternative form of family building, rather than as
infertility treatments. These alternatives have complex psychosocial
implications. A recent book, *Beyond Infertility: The New Paths to
Parenthood* by Susan Cooper and Ellen Glazer, provides a comprehensive look at the issues involved in ovum donation, donor insemination, surrogacy, gestational care, and embryo adoption. Guid-
ance in explaining these methods of family building to children is
found in *The Flight of the Stork: What Children Think (and When)
about Sex and Family Building* by Anne Bernstein.

One-Child Resolution

Reassessing a desired family size requires confronting your fantasy of the expected family, mourning its loss, and then reevaluating the status quo. This holds true whenever the existing family size differs from what was originally planned. This process is markedly different from that of ending treatment and feeling defeated by the process. Affirming the family as it is requires a conscious decision based on positive motivations. When couples choose not to adopt, they have the means to increase their family but elect not to, preferring that the family remain as is. Similarly, some decide to forgo treatment, preferring to invest their energy in the child they have.

Many parents have a natural ambivalence about having another child, wondering whether they can ever love another child as much as their firstborn or whether they can handle caring for another. Those who have experienced secondary infertility have additional questions to consider in deciding whether to continue or cease trying to increase their family:

Facing IVF, I have been having confused thoughts on having another baby. Should I or shouldn't I? Am I too old now (thirty-nine)? Is my husband (forty-three)? Is my boy too old to enjoy a close relationship with a sibling (nine)? Will it be too hard to accept a newborn into our lifestyle? Will it be odd taking another child to school in five or six years and seeing all the younger mothers? Is it better to just leave our family as is and not ruffle the waters? Am I opening Pandora's box? Will the baby be healthy? What if I have triplets? How will we pay off the bill, which will surely total over $23,000?

Deciding to discontinue treatment and relinquish the dream of having another child is not easy, as the following vignette illustrates; however, positive feelings may gradually coexist with the negative ones and may in time predominate:

Gradually, I'm coming to grips with this, and I have been trying to focus on the wonderful times we have with our daughter and the things that we can do as a family of three that bigger families cannot. At the same time, I can still get teary-eyed when I see a newborn, or jealous of families with two or three kids.

As Jean and Michael Carter write in *Sweet Grapes: How to Stop Being Infertile and Start Living Again,*

> There is hope that you can no longer be infertile without necessarily being fertile.... Infertility is a negative concept.... Being infertile means defining your life according to the loss of your fertility.... The alternative to infertility—that is, the alternative to defining your life according to what you don't have—is to define your life according to what you do have and can have.[5]

The next history reflects this understanding and shows how someone moved beyond being infertile to being content as the mother of one:

> I desperately wanted to have another child. Our daughter is now four years old, and about two years ago, I decided this desperate need of mine . . . was not going to ruin my life. Infertility is horrid! . . . Today I have come to the realization that I may never have another child. I've learned to accept that reality and say, "That's OK." . . . There are also a lot of advantages in having one child—and I look to all the positive aspects of that. For one thing, she gets an incredible amount of attention; . . . typically, an only child is very smart . . . due to all this attention.... Our house is nice and peaceful with just the three of us.... Also, by having an only child, we're able to afford a lot more for her. We'll plan to send her to the best college. This summer I traveled with her and my mother, visiting fifteen states—and we had a great time! I could not have done this with more than one child. . . . I could not have tolerated children fighting while I was driving over 6,000 miles! . . . Now, having a four-year-old, I have my freedom again. I have time to do lots of personal activities, . . . while I'm still able to be a full-time mother at home.

Pregnancy and Single and Multiple Births after Secondary Infertility

Pregnancy achieved after infertility often brings anxieties along with the joy. After all, couples are now painfully aware that things can and do go wrong. If an earlier pregnancy was a source of unmitigated happiness, this newfound worry may seem to be another loss, the loss of peace of mind. The longed-for pregnancy that was fantasized as recapturing the earlier experience is in reality a different one. Each pregnancy is unique, even without infertility, and a pregnant mother may find that her status is primarily that of a mother, with the specialness of pregnancy being somewhat eclipsed. Women may want to savor the experience after trying so long to become pregnant, yet now find that their other responsibilities and worries diminish it. As one woman writes,

> A downside [of being an infertility patient] is I am not quite trusting that this is real and that . . . I will have a baby. Although I never had a miscarriage, I was really worried in the beginning, and even now every twinge that I feel is a concern. I cannot wait to hold this son of mine.

Although many couples eventually are able to become pregnant and give birth to another child, this does not represent the end of their reproductive lives. The experience of having been infertile continues to shape family-planning decisions:

> I had been fitted for a diaphragm and intended to use it for a while. Maybe it was our increased feeling of vulnerability . . . , maybe it was a feeling that we were unlikely to get pregnant even if we tried, maybe it was just general recklessness, but we did not consistently use birth control and I found myself pregnant when [my baby] was four months old—I thought the book *The Long Awaited Stork* put it best when it said that in this situation, you would probably feel both burdened and blessed! I tell people this must be what it's like for normal people—to lose track of where you are in your cycle—to have ambivalent feelings about being pregnant—to just get pregnant without "trying."

Just as past fertility is no guarantee of future fertility, so past infertility does not necessarily mean future infertility. Regaining control of reproduction is an important goal.

Some couples find that the pregnancy they achieve following infertility treatment may not be the long-hoped-for repeat of their first pregnancy, but rather a multiple pregnancy, with its particular concerns.

It is not uncommon for parents who may have been trying to achieve an "ideal" family of two children to find themselves instead giving birth to multiples. Since couples are often pessimistic about their chances of becoming pregnant at all, the news of twins or higher multiples almost always comes as a shock, despite the statistics about the effects of fertility drugs. Ironically, the same parents who were concerned about their child lacking a sibling now worry that the child must adjust to being the oldest of three or more children.

> I told myself during the secondary infertility treatments that in part I was doing it for my son. I wanted very much for him to haver a brother or sister. Yet now that I'm expecting twins, I fear it may have a negative effect on him. One baby would be a big adjustment for him, but two will be even more so. I worry that my attention and patience will be limited. So there is guilt, now and before this pregnancy. I have been sick a great deal in the past year due to surgery, medications, and now morning sickness. And I question if I'm being a good enough parent.

As mentioned previously, there are no ideal family forms, and it may be the parents' feelings that determine how the child accepts the additional siblings. After what may have been a prolonged period of being a single child, he or she may find it hard to share parents with more than one baby. A slightly older first child may, however, be better able to accept the arrival of twins and all the attention they receive.

Many couples experience conceiving twins as a bonus for their efforts and feel that parenting multiples is no hardship compared with infertility treatment. But for others, although they do feel blessed, they may also feel once again out of control at having once again been unable to determine their family size. An uncomfortable or high-risk multiple pregnancy deprives them of a chance to relive the former pregnancy and instead presents them with a new and potentially frightening situation.

The announcement of a multiple pregnancy is almost always responded to with congratulations, and couples may feel guilty acknowledging any ambivalent feelings, even to themselves. After all, they sorely wanted another child—how can they be distressed with more than they bargained for? While couples have been told the odds of having multiples, most are surprised by the news: Getting pregnant at all seems so remote that the idea of having multiples is not taken seriously.

Even fewer couples expect to give birth to triplets or higher multiples. While statistically there is not a high probability of this (about 5 percent for Assisted Reproductive Technology (ART) procedures),[6] this is a possibility that needs to be considered. Families with higher multiples confront numerous challenges, including premature delivery, low birth weights, and subsequent depletion of financial and emotional resources. Couples who feel they would be unable to deal with higher multiples should discuss this with their physician as part of their medical decision-making process. Caution could be taken with medications, fewer embryos reimplanted in ART procedures, and the risks and advantages of multifetal reduction discussed in case the situation arises. This controversial procedure in which the number of fetuses is reduced in order to increase the likelihood of the survival of the remaining fetuses raises both medical and emotional issues. This procedure is discussed at length in *Beyond Infertility: The New Paths to Parenthood* by Susan Cooper and Ellen Glazer.

A multiple pregnancy raises questions of how much to share concerning the infertility treatments when strangers ask how the multiple pregnancy was achieved. Parents don't owe the public the recipe for their success. Rather they should decide and do what is most comfortable for their family. Resources, such as the National Mothers of Twins organization and *TWINS* magazine, are available to aid those parenting multiples.

Parenting after Secondary Infertility

As cited above, Ellen Glazer's *The Long-Awaited Stork: A Guide to Parenting after Infertility* describes the special dynamics of parenting after infertility. Chapter 7 of this book details parents' singular feelings toward their child while experiencing secondary infertility. For those parents who do go on to have another child, either through birth or adoption, the question then becomes, Do they parent any differently from how they did previously?

Many factors influence this outcome: whether the secondary infertility was recurring or first-time, the spacing of the siblings, and the specific events leading to the child's arrival into the family. But a major difference between parenting after primary vs. secondary infertility is that those in the latter group are experienced parents. It is commonly accepted that parents, having raised a child, are more relaxed, and for many, this tendency may outweigh the dynamics of parenting after infertility, while for others the specialness of the conception, adoption, or memory of pregnancy losses may predominate.

Moving toward Resolution

As parents coping with secondary infertility, you may be particularly motivated to resolve your crisis. You realize the effects of your struggle on your children and want to be able to enjoy them completely. You feel the passage of time as you see your child mature. The majority of parents are not inclined to drift, but rather spend a limited period intensely exploring all alternatives. At some point, you may feel that the desire to reclaim your lives is even stronger than your desire for another child. Some spouses find that they actually cross paths, with one deciding to go forward just as the other is beginning to wind down. Good communication is crucial to reaching an outcome acceptable to you both; in some cases, a third party is useful to facilitate communication and decision making. What is important is that a resolution is reached so that you and your family can get on with your lives. Infertility for some of you will remain a part of your lives—but fortunately, it will cease to feel like it is dominating your whole lives.

10

Surviving Secondary Infertility

I am living my life again now.
—Woman following secondary infertility

The potentially devastating effects of secondary infertility are well known to you if you have experienced it or worked with those who have. Less apparent is that you will survive it. Unfortunately, there are no shortcuts or magic solutions. Grieving the loss of the child you haven't had is the surest (but hardest) path to resolution. While it may be scary to think about painful subjects, there's no way to resolve the pain without experiencing it. This chapter describes what has helped others cope with secondary infertility. While no single remedy is right for everyone, everyone needs to have some resources for coping. There are strategies to help counter many of the feelings caused by the infertility: isolation, grief, loss of control, and an inability to get on with life. The following account describes how one woman now awaiting on international adoption utilized supports to help her:

> I feel like I have been on an emotional rollercoaster for the past five years. . . . When I look back, I feel I've come a long way. . . . Counseling has been most helpful to me over the past three years; . . . it has really kept me together. . . . [Also,] involvement with RESOLVE—attending some monthly meetings and small get-togethers—realizing there are other people in the same boat. . . . My husband's realization that I had a right to my feelings and the support he has learned to provide me with [helped me to cope]. . . . I am able to now talk openly about my infertility and not get upset with people prodding and prying. I can accept that I will probably not conceive ever again. I just hope with all my heart that this adoption will work out.

Grieving as a Path to Resolution

Grieving is painful, difficult work, acknowledging that there has been a loss. Remaining hopeful and positive while worrying that the treatments may not work is an arduous emotional feat. Alternating between such anticipatory grieving and the hopefulness experienced during treatment leads to the emotional rollercoaster of infertility.

Some, thinking grieving is an admission of defeat, suppress these feelings, and operate on the assumption that "everything will work out." But losses have already been experienced: loss of control, a sense of failure, repeated disappointments, and a feeling of having been left behind. Yet it is possible to grieve for all that you have already gone through without abandoning the dream of another biological child. Couples who do have successful pregnancies feel their grieving was a worthwhile part of gaining perspective on their infertility. Similarly, couples who complete their families through adoption realize that grieving for their lost fertility enabled them to move ahead and actualize their desire to parent:

> Much of our healing has taken place through the adoption of our second daughter—now three years old. . . . It is so much different than giving birth, and I did grieve the loss of being able to be pregnant. And yet, we have another child!

You and your partner may be in different stages of the grieving process. It is hard to grieve alone. Being unsupported is scary and may cause you to question your perceptions. According to Jean and Michael Carter, authors of *Sweet Grapes: How to Stop Being Infertile and Start Living Again*:

> For an infertile couple, grieving must be a mutual act. They must allow for real communication, even if it does hurt, to eventually get out of the denial phase. . . . Facing loss is what we call mourning. . . . [I]t's okay to mourn, to feel the despair, hopelessness, and even depression that comes with the loss. . . . [I]t is through this awareness of loss that we come to accept it, to make peace with it. . . . However long it is, though, most people eventually find that they have come to accept the loss.[1]

For many couples, infertility is the first loss they must grieve. Most people fear grieving; they are afraid that it will be unending, that they will bottom out and never recover. Fortunately, this is not the case. Those who have coped with the loss of a loved one may experience similar emotions and go through similar stages of the grieving process. While the infertility can reactivate earlier feelings of loss, they have the advantage of knowing that their grief will diminish over time.

Human beings are generally resilient and seem to have an automatic shut-off valve to keep themselves from being overwhelmed by more pain than they can handle. Temporary denial can be protective, allowing the grief to be experienced gradually. You might not recognize that you have been undergoing a grieving process, because the grief is diffused and not focused on a single loss. Often couples feel that they are not moving any closer to resolution, only to suddenly realize that they are actually in a different and more comfortable place. Grief in its acute stages is finite; people can go from their lowest point in years to suddenly being ready to move on. It is as though the grief has finally burned itself out. Often, however, it is a less dramatic progression.

Once you acknowledge the loss, you can mourn and begin healing. Healing can't be rushed, though, and many people despair that they will always feel unhappy and stuck in the middle of resolving their feelings:

> It is true that the passage of time heals. It is also true that it can't be hurried or telescoped. Time seems to bring with it a sense of *perspective* or "the larger view" of life for those who have had tunnel vision focused on infertility for a number of years. When feelings have been properly worked through, they tend to subside and a kind of *selective remembering* often takes place so that the really painful memories and events are muted. Time is a healer, time is a friend. But *time takes time.*[2]

This does not mean that feelings of loss go away entirely; rather, as the following brief vignette reflects, they are muted:

> No. we aren't without pain, and still have moments of tears. We have learned that grief is never completely done, but less intense as time goes by. We get frustrated by others' remarks, but are more apt to make a civil reply instead of blowing up at them or becoming a puddle of tears.

As parents, you may be particularly motivated to resolve your grief and get on with your lives. Perhaps your fantasies about families have been linked to the spacing of your children. You may see your child getting older and realize how much infertility has overshadowed your enjoyment of that child's life. In some ways, the grieving process of those undergoing secondary infertility is intensified because of the perceived time constraints; however, the awareness of the passage of time can also serve to facilitate letting go and moving on.

You may find that your desire for another child diminishes over time. For instance, if you wanted to have children close together in age, you may find that a new baby will conflict with the life you have established. Reassessing your goals, given your current realities, does not negate your earlier desire for another child. Once your child is in school, you may begin to see the positive side of not having anymore children. Your concerns about raising a single child may lessen as your child becomes more involved with peers. With the passage of time, you may become ready to reinvest yourself in a career.

Judith Calica, a clinical social worker and longtime RESOLVE volunteer, points out the need for couples to reassess their family planning decisions as time goes on. She explains that, following infertility, some couples don't use contraception, reasoning that they would be grateful for a miracle. However, the optimal time for their having another child can pass without their rethinking earlier contraceptive decisions. Using contraception after infertility may seem unnecessary. However, ironically, some formerly infertile couples find themselves unhappily pregnant at a time in their lives when they cannot deal with another child.

When the depression surrounding the infertility lifts and the "tunnel vision" lessens, you may become able to appreciate the other parts of your life that have been eclipsed by the infertility, including your family as it is:

> Slowly, slowly, I began to accept this condition. I fought it for so long, not believing it could have happened to me. I am living my life again now. It was a terrible, terrible struggle, but now I can concentrate on what I *do* have, a wonderful, fourteen-year-old, healthy, happy son who gives me much love and happiness. I also realize how lucky I am to

have such a wonderful husband. He really stood by me through this harrowing ordeal. I know he also is hurt by our inability to have more children, but he has proved over and over that he loves me enough to endure it with me.

Finding Support

Few natural support networks exist for those of you experiencing secondary infertility. The importance of finding others who can understand and validate your feelings cannot be overstated. For some, it is vital to have supportive doctors and nurses; others are fortunate to have supportive spouses, family, and friends. Most, however, eventually feel the need for additional support. It may seem odd to seek support from strangers, except for the powerful bond between those sharing a common struggle. It is imperative that you "find someone who understands what you are going through, since just talking about it helps." Many people have found professional counseling helpful, and a combination of counseling and peer support is frequently recommended:

> I think that going to group counseling with other women experiencing secondary infertility was the best support for me. Not only was the counseling helpful, but more importantly, it put me in touch with a wonderful group of friends who have been able to provide the support and friendship that I need. I also saw a counselor individually for a few sessions, which was also helpful. . . . Find a support group. There are other women out there going through the same thing, and it is so therapeutic to have the support from people who are feeling the same things that you are. They are the ones who can really understand.

> Somehow I coped and found RESOLVE. . . . That organization is a godsend, and I can't say enough good about it. They cover everything involved with treatment and also alternative ways to build a family.

> PLEASE stress in your book how important one or both of these [counseling and support groups] are. It is nice to feel that you are not alone and that, others can truly understand your feelings. I have mentioned to my support group that when I am with them, I am most at peace with my situation. I do not have to explain myself or justify my feelings.

And again:

> RESOLVE—participating in a support group run by a social worker therapist has been the most helpful. Being with four other women who have experienced similar feelings, and feeling free to express some of the outrageous thoughts I've had, was freeing. It was comforting to be with people who did not judge. The experience of the group helped me gain perspective.

RESOLVE groups for mothers experiencing infertility are powerful, filled with some tears and much laughter, recognition, and acceptance.

It is unfortunate that only a small percentage of those experiencing secondary infertility affiliate with RESOLVE. National staff report that a membership survey reveals that only 3 to 5 percent of their members classify themselves as secondarily infertile, despite the fact that this group constitutes the majority of the infertile population. Some of the reasons for this disparity are discussed in Chapter 5, "Caught between Two Worlds." The current national executive director of RESOLVE, Inc., Diane Aronson, laments this trend: "Services exist within RESOLVE which could be of tremendous benefit to this group and to which they are most welcome and entitled. It is important that RESOLVE be seen as an organization serving and advocating for all of the infertile population, not only the childless infertile."

Even if there is no RESOLVE chapter in your area, you can still benefit from the RESOLVE network. The organization has a Member-to-Member contact system that provides a vehicle for giving and receiving peer support. In addition, the newsletter runs "Requests for Contact." One member from Israel writes to the newsletter about the response to her earlier letter:

> I am writing to thank you. When I submitted a Request for Contact in the National Newsletter, I did not imagine the response that I would receive. . . . Most of the women who wrote . . . shared their problems, treatments, frustrations and pain. For the first time since my miscarriage four years ago, I feel less alone. There are women I can turn to who will listen and understand and never get fed up because they are or have been where I am. Thank you RESOLVE for giving me access to this caring network.[3]

Redefining Success

While speaking of "giving up" or "quitting" treatment has negative connotations of failure, "reclaiming your lives" and "enjoying the existing family" represent successful outcomes. You may need to redefine success and achievement in terms other than fertility: Resolving a major life crisis is an important achievement, just as getting on with your lives is a vital measure of success. Discontinuing treatment, which may feel like "giving up," can in truth be a courageous decision validating your lives.

Mourning losses allows people to refocus on affirmative possibilities. A qualitative difference exists between (a) accepting one's loss and (b) reevaluating one's life and seeing the positives in the status quo. Just as the meanings of *childless* and *child-free* reflect the difference between a loss and a positive outcome, so too is there a difference between seeing the advantages of your family as it is and settling for a family size you feel is incomplete.

The premise of *Sweet Grapes: How to Stop Being Infertile and Start Living Again* is that there is a potential for gain with loss, that all situations can be seen as having positive and negative aspects. The following quotation has been adapted to apply to the secondarily infertile, as opposed to those considering child-free living:

> Infertility is a negative concept . . . characterized by wanting what you don't have—[another] biological child, of course. Being infertile means defining your life according to the loss of your fertility. . . . [W]e offer the alternative of no longer infertile, or no longer actively infertile. We don't want to imply, however, that your loss simply vanished. It will always be there. It is an important part of who you are. Instead, no longer infertile means that in the loss of your fertility you can find the potential for gain. The alternative to infertility . . . is to define your life according to what you do have and can have.[4]

> We could make a choice. . . . Of course, there was still some final grieving to do. Hope is hard to give up, even when it has become more painful than helpful. . . . We did have a choice. . . . [W]e could . . . [define] our lives by what we lack or we could . . . [affirm] the potential gain that comes of living without [as many children as desired]. . . . Instead of being unsuccessful parents-to be, we were very successful [parents]. Failure was no longer the major theme of our lives.[5]

As parents experiencing infertility, you can focus on your success as parents, rather than on your failure to have additional children. This may require you to rethink what makes a successful parent, if you feel you have failed your child by not producing a sibling:

> The number of children you have doesn't mean you're a great mom, or a real woman; it's the love you give to your child. Your child is precious; give that child all the love you had to give to all the children you wanted.

You may find that although you would never willingly have experienced infertility, it has had some positive consequences:

> It has been over six years since we started to conceive again. We have no miracle pregnancy to speak of in glowing terms, and our lives have taken off in some unexpected directions. We like who we have become, though we don't like the way in which it came about. We have become more sensitive, less apt to be walked over, and better able to speak up for the things that we need. My husband and I are also quite thankful that our low points have never occurred at the same time. We are better able to understand and share in the grief of others.

A quote in *Sweet Grapes: How to Stop Being Infertile and Start Living Again* illustrates that infertilite individuals can think of themselves as survivors rather than victims.

> All those hours of communication have built two people who know how to talk to each other and also know how important it is to take the time to talk with each other. Yes, our self-esteem was tremendously battered by our infertility, but it was also rebuilt as we learned to deal with the crisis as a couple and as individuals. We now see ourselves as crisis managers and as survivors. . . . We know that we can allow ourselves to grieve and that we can handle the emotional impact of problems. We see ourselves as strong people who can work through difficulties. We have also learned how important it is to keep the various aspects of our lives in balance as we face different ages and stages. Our infertility helped us create a strong marriage unit that we use and enjoy every day of our lives.[6]

Informing and Empowering Yourselves

It seems that at some point during the infertility struggle, you may no longer be looking so much for a successful pregnancy as for some understanding of your infertility. Lacking an answer as to why you are no longer able to conceive or carry to term makes the loss even harder to accept. Answers, when available, help to make the loss more absolute, more comprehensible, and therefore easier to grieve. Many couples with secondary infertility fall into the unexplained category, a status that can make it very hard to move on.

As devastating as it is to receive an absolute diagnosis, at least there is an answer, and future options are clearer. Feeling that your doctor has done everything possible and having participated actively in the decision making make it easier to end treatment; if you feel that you have not received adequate treatment and that you should have been more involved, you might be plagued with regrets. (See Chapter 8, "Working with Your Medical Providers.")

When respondents to the survey for this book were asked their advice for others experiencing secondary infertility, caveats about medical care were a strong, recurring theme: "Research the doctor and clinic very well. Just because it's in a respected university doesn't always mean the treatment is appropriate or adequate." In retrospect, another realizes, "I strongly feel that I relinquished much of my treatment options to my physicians, who I thought were more on top of my case than they appear to have been. I would be a more vocal advocate on my own behalf." One woman reports that the hardest part of her infertility was being misdiagnosed, being put on fertility drugs, and having her condition made worse; she laments that the doctor "wasted months of my reproductive life and probably cost me the chance of my most wanted baby." Speaking from her experience, she tells others:

> Go to a reproductive endocrinologist at the first sign of difficulty. Get a second opinion. Read. Research. Read some more! Don't wait to seek medical care. See your problem as a failure of medicine to diagnose and treat you. Don't see yourself as a failure. Infertility is a symptom of a medical problem.
>
> Do not be intimidated by your doctor. Keep a chart of your own with every . . . visit. Buy a bound notebook and keep a log of your monthly visits—what was discussed . . . , who you saw, what drugs you took. Record interactions with office staff. Think about what your expectations are at each visit, and communicate your expectations to M.D.s/staff.

Participating actively in your care is empowering, restoring some degree of control and making the infertility more manageable and less overwhelming. Becoming knowledgeable helped many respondents cope with their infertility because it was something concrete they could do and thus made them feel less passive. Becoming informed and advocating for yourself are vital in coming to terms with the infertility, regardless of outcome:

> I informed myself—I read as many books and articles as I could on infertility, and it helped because our local doctors didn't communicate well. I pushed to see a specialist; at least now I feel listened to and acknowledged, even if they never find a problem.

Getting Unstuck: Need for Closure

Some treatment decisions are based not so much on the likelihood of a successful pregnancy as on your need to do everything possible to achieve closure. One woman explains that she "couldn't stop treatment until I'd done all I could do." Although she "felt at the end of line," she was also beginning to see that she could be happy once it was all over. A final medical consultation with another doctor can reassure you that everything appropriate has been tried. What constitutes a fair trial is subjective, and many patients today extend treatment way beyond what would have been recommended even five or ten years ago.

The lack of fertility is baffling, and cannot be solved by using traditional problem-solving approaches. You can do everything right and still be unable to achieve the desired result. Being unable to control the outcome through your efforts is a new experience for many couples. One woman relates her frustration at being out-of-control:

> The lack of control is the most frustrating. I have an "achiever" personality. I have always set goals and plans for myself and have always attained them. This is one plan which I cannot fulfill, and it has nothing to do with me. I have done everything I can do, and it is outside of my control. Letting go of the monthly hoping has also been difficult for me; I still feel very hopeful before my period each month, then very sad when I find that I am not pregnant. After four years of trying, one would think that this rollercoaster would stop and the hopefulness would lessen. But for some reason, I have not been able to do this, and

the monthly rollercoaster is very draining emotionally. Lastly, it is very difficult to deal with the fact that sometimes the emotions just unexpectedly creep to the surface, and a fleeting comment, a new baby, or a pregnant woman can bring me to tears. I do not like this lack of control. These incidents are becoming fewer, but they still surprise me at times, and this is very frustrating.

Deciding to stop treatment is one way of regaining control. You need to make a conscious decision about options, rather than drifting or remaining in limbo. Couples commonly articulate that the pain and hardship of undergoing advanced reproductive technology are nothing compared with the pain of admitting that treatment has not worked:

> The hardest part will be finally giving up and stopping treatment. An analogy might be an athletic challenge like running a race . . . and never being able to run it again. . . . I think that as infertility treatment proceeds for a woman, the desire (or drive) gets greater and greater. By that, I mean that as the treatment becomes more complex, . . . the infertile couple becomes more and more compulsive and determined to achieve [fertility].

Even ceasing aggressive treatment does not take away all of the hope. This can be a mixed blessing. Some couples decide to use contraception to eliminate "that little bit of hope each month, . . . enough hope . . . to hurt." Contraception can be a "declaration of independence from the cycle of hope and despair."[7] One woman took steps to end the ambiguity and create an absolute status by having her tubes surgically closed, thus regaining control and removing the hurt of hopefulness:

> In the beginning of treatment, . . . I said we'd put an endpoint of my fortieth birthday for trying to conceive. As it neared, I felt more "iffy" and wanted to try for "just one more month," but we held to the deadline. And for me, that meant really stopping trying, so I had a tubal ligation. This gave me a sense of control and ended the monthly disappointment. It's been over a year now since my tubal ligation, and I'm feeling much more settled in my life. Now that I know *this* is my family, I'm feeling OK about raising a child without brothers and sisters. I'm seeing real positive things about our life now—how much fun we have and the neat things we can do.

While most couples will not go to this length to achieve closure, it is important to reach a similar point of resolution and peace.

Establishing Rituals

Rituals are useful to mark important life events and transitions: weddings, funerals, even baby showers. There are no recognized rituals for unacknowledged losses such as infertility or even pregnancy loss. Few people receive condolence notes or flowers following a miscarriage. Some couples have decided to develop their own meaningful ways of memorializing the children they had hoped to have: Some write letters to the unborn children, plant a tree or make a donation in their memory, or hold memorial services. These rituals can be helpful in achieving closure and provide an avenue for others to respond to your loss.

On the other hand, rituals can joyfully mark the decision to get on with your lives. Celebrating the decision to accept and affirm your family as is, or to proceed with an alternative such as adoption, is a concrete way to mark this milestone and to let others know of your status. A family holiday or party to enjoy your existing family or while awaiting an adoption is a positive way to mark the end of what has most likely been a difficult time and the start of the next stage of your family life.

A symbolic act marking the decision to affirm your family as it is can be to give away baby equipment that has been saved for the next child. This process is trying, but some find it to be cathartic and ultimately liberating. Some couples try to manage the task in a way that is meaningful: giving the baby paraphernalia to charity or to a friend who is finally pregnant after infertility. You may have strong feelings about relatives to whom you would prefer or *not* prefer to pass on these personal items. And, you may decide to store precious keepsakes, which, once out of sight, can later be treasured for what they were, rather than causing pain for how they were not used.

Living Life Apart from Infertility

An insidious aspect of infertility is its tendency to take over your life—it is hard to contain. Infertility is not just a medical problem; it also creeps into every aspect of daily life. It is difficult but important to try to maintain a sense of who you are, separate from the infertility. I am constantly impressed by the range of strengths and abilities that I see in couples who fail to appreciate the positives about themselves because they feel so defeated by their infertility. Talents and career successes are often devalued because they are not fertility-related. But when your self-esteem has been battered by infertility, it is particularly important to have other sources of gratification in order to feel good about yourself.

One woman explains how she shared her journal and poetry with her doctor so that he would know her "as a whole person." She also found it helpful to buy a "beautiful new wardrobe and *dress up* . . . to go to the clinic." She treated herself to a trip to New York City and "had a blast." Others recommend writing, painting your feelings, talking about infertility to "safe people," working, and going out. In short, don't put your life on hold. Some enjoy pursuing hobbies, exercising, learning a new skill, or taking a class. Again, the choice of outlet is personal and idiosyncratic; what is universal is the need to have some activities that help you feel good about yourself. A guide to coping with pregnancy loss recommends:

> Try to get involved with outside interests. Pregnancy loss and infertility treatments can become all-consuming. Other activities can be a welcome distraction and can also help you discover creative outlets and develop potential in other areas.[8]

One hazard of infertility is that often individuals feel stymied in every aspect of their lives. Women can't even buy clothing without wondering whether they will be pregnant; decisions about vacations are often put on hold; buying a minivan or a house with too many bedrooms can be a painful reminder of unfulfilled fantasies.

Career limbo can also result; just at a time when you might otherwise be going ahead with your career, your life is on hold. You might keep an unsatisfactory job for the flexibility that comes from having worked in the same place for a while. Others may feel that taking a new job is not fair to a new employer, since they hope to become pregnant soon. And many men and women cannot risk losing insurance benefits with a job shift. You may feel too depleted to fight the inertia and comfort of what is known to tackle new challenges. In this way, many are deprived of work satisfaction that might to some degree offset the feelings of failure from the infertility.

One woman insightfully details the interrelationships between her infertility and job frustrations:

> I find that when I'm really suffering with this infertility, work becomes more burdensome. It sometimes feels like such a waste of time. My heart tells me I should be home with a baby, not struggling with all these seemingly burdensome and meaningless tasks. This . . . has more to do with the incredible amount of energy that an ongoing crisis takes, leaving little for other areas of my life. Sometimes it feels like trying to get pregnant is a part-time job: visiting various doctors, reading materials, going to meetings, and, worst of all, fighting my insurance company for coverage. And finally, it affects my work in terms of career. For two years, I have put off looking for another job because "What if I get pregnant? I can't be pregnant on a new job! I'll need all the vacation and sick time I've accumulated over the years on this job!" or "How can I expect a new boss to allow me the time off I need for all these infertility appointments? Etc." On the one hand, I stay because it's easier to cope when my job is one I am used to and know so well. Yet on the other hand, moving on to another job could be a healthy distraction from infertility. And maybe I wouldn't feel so stuck, a feeling that is so like the one created by infertility.

Of course, your existing child is an obvious source of gratification, although the experience can be bittersweet, as has been discussed in Chapter 7:

> I tried to focus on enjoying the family I had and not let infertility destroy my happiness there. I tried to take my son to the park, swimming, and on other outings (even when I didn't really want to), and it was always fun for both of us.

Many people find relief from the stresses of infertility through various relaxation techniques, such as meditation, self-hypnosis, visualization, positive imagery, and even acupuncture. Aline Zoldbrod has written a useful pamphlet *Getting Around the Boulder in the Road: Using Imagery to Cope with Fertility Problems*. The use of antidepressants, which could alleviate some of the emotional pain of infertility, is rare because of the reluctance to use medications while trying to conceive.

Searching for Meaning

Spirituality

Just as the infertility crisis can cause you to question your relationship with one another and with family and friends, so too can it lead to a crisis of faith. "Bad things" aren't supposed to "happen to good people," as Rabbi Kushner addresses in his popular book. For others, spirituality provides a source of strength and gives meaning to their suffering. The following account traces the questioning and finally the answer that religion provided to a couple following an ectopic pregnancy:

> We were heartbroken and again questioned why—myself to the point of apologizing to my husband and believing it was completely my fault. God later revealed to me that it is not for me to question why but to trust in Him and walk with Him and let Him carry me through this most difficult, heartbreaking experience. . . . My only solution has been to trust God, and He has faithfully blessed me in that trust. . . . The Lord blessed us with a beautiful healthy boy within six weeks after [we] first contact[ed] our attorney. We know that adoption was the route God had for us and that our son is truly God's miracle in our lives.

Some find comfort in the idea that their infertility is not random or meaningless, but part of a larger plan:

> I have read the Bible, and through the church sermons I have realized this is not my main purpose in life—to have children. I am thankful for my salvation through Jesus, and this is the most important thing. The Bible never promised an easy life or anything you want. I have to look at what I can do for the world. . . .
>
> I do know God is faithful and he will not forsake us. He has a plan for us, and I just have to patiently wait for that plan to come to fruition in His time.

This woman, while perhaps waiting patiently, was not waiting passively; rather, she was considering both donor insemination and adoption. Many women reason that treatment and alternatives are also part of God's plan.

Helping Others

Some individuals try to make meaning out of their suffering through helping others in a similar situation. One member of a RE-SOLVE support group, after "graduating" from the group, went on to start discussion groups for others in her area. She also appeared on a national talk show to focus attention on secondary infertility. Others write letters to the editor in support of insurance coverage, advocate with legislators, or take on the task of educating others about infertility. Some volunteer for the local RESOLVE chapter.

Many of those who shared their stories for this book did so out of a desire to help others in the same situation. The wish to create something positive out of an unwanted crisis helps the helper to gain perspective, as well as aiding those who are currently experiencing the crisis: "If I can ease one person's pain by sharing mine, then mine will have not been in vain. In helping others I help myself as well.[9] Finally, as one woman wrote, "It is very difficult to put such personal feelings on paper and submit them to a stranger, but it is my hope that by doing so, others may read your book and find some support."

Appendix

Survey

1. Age and Age of Partner

2. Age of Child[ren]

3. Did you have difficulty conceiving previously? If so, what was your diagnosis and treatment?

4. At what point did you seek treatment for secondary infertility? From ob/gyn or specialist?

5. Do/did you have a diagnosis? If so, what?

6. Do you think your prior fertility influenced your diagnosis and/or treatment? For instance, did you or your doctor make any assumptions based on your past fertility?

7. If you experienced infertility previously, how did it feel to find yourself dealing with it again? How would you compare the experiences of primary/secondary infertility?

8. If you had no difficulty conceiving earlier, how did it feel to find yourself dealing with infertility?

9. How do you think your experience differs from that of the childless infertile?

10. How have others reacted to your infertility? Have family, friends, and/or co-workers been supportive?

11. Do you feel the fact that you have a child[ren] influences people's reactions? If so, in what way?

12. Have you discussed the infertility with your child? If so, what did you say? If not, do you think s/he knows?

13. Does your child[ren] express feelings about having a sibling? If so, how does that affect you?

14. How do you combine treatment with parenting? Have you ever taken your child with you to doctor's appointments?

15. How has the infertility affected you emotionally? Socially? At work?

16. How would you compare your reactions to those of your partner?

17. Has infertility affected your relationship with your partner?

18. Has it affected your relationship with your child[ren] and/or your ability to parent? Do you feel they have been affected in other ways?

19. Has the infertility affected your involvement in child-oriented activities?

20. What has helped you to cope with the infertility?

21. What are some of your reasons for wanting another child? What are some of your partner's reasons?

22. Are you exploring any of the following: adoption? donor insemination or donor ovum? a one child family? If so, what factors are influencing your decision making?

23. What are your feelings about "only" children? What do you see as the public perception of "only" children?

24. How many siblings do you and your partner have? How do you get along with them?

25. What is your vision of an "ideal" family size? Why?

26. If you have given birth or adopted following secondary infertility, what has that been like for your family?

27. What has been the hardest part of experiencing secondary infertility for you? for your partner?

28. What would you like others to realize about secondary infertility?

29. What would you like to say to others experiencing secondary infertility?

30. Please add any additional comments.

THANK YOU FOR YOUR HELP!

Resources

Organizations

Adoptive Families of America, the largest organization for adoptive parents in the world, which provides referrals to local parent groups.
>3333 Hwy 100 North
>Minneapolis, MN 55422
>612-537-0316

American Fertility Society (AFS), an international association of professionals with a special interest in fertility.
>1209 Montgomery Highway
>Birmingham, AL. 35216-2809
>315-724-4348

National Council for Adoption, an adoption advocacy organization with referrals to member agencies for traditional, confidential adoptions.
>1930 17th Street NW
>Washington, D.C. 20009
>202-328-1200

Parents of Only Children, an organization promoting communication among only children, their parents, spouses and friends, and professionals dedicated to influencing societal attitudes toward only children.
>4719 Reed Road
>Suite 121
>Columbus, OH. 43220
>614-442-0873

RESOLVE, Inc., national infertility organization providing education, support, and advocacy services with chapters nationwide.
>1310 Broadway
>Somerville, MA. 02144-1731
>Business Office 617-623-1156
>HelpLine 617-623-0744

Recommended Readings

Bernstein, Anne. *The Flight of the Stork: What Children Think (and When) about Sex and Family Building*, Revised Edition. Indianapolis: Perspectives Press, 1994.

Bombardieri, Merle. *The Baby Decision: How to Make the Most Important Choice of Your Life*. New York: Rawson Wade, 1981.

Carter, Jean and Michael Carter. *Sweet Grapes: How to Stop being Infertile and Start Living Again*. Indianapolis: Perspectives Press, 1989.

Cooper, Susan and Ellen Glazer. *Beyond Infertility: The New Paths to Parenthood*. New York: Lexington Books, 1994.

Gilman, Lois. *The Adoption Resource Book*. New York: Harper Collins, rev. 1992.

Glazer, Ellen. *The Long-Awaited Stork: A Guide to Parenting after Infertility*. Lexington, MA.: Lexington Books, 1990.

Ellen Glazer and Susan Cooper. *Without Child: Experiencing and Resolving Infertility*. Lexington, MA.: Lexington Books, 1988.

Harkness, Carla. *The Infertility Book: A Comprehensive Medical and Emotional Guide*, Second Edition. Berkeley: Celestial Arts, 1992.

Johnston, Patricia Irwin. *Taking Charge of Infertility*. Indianapolis: Perspectives Press, 1994.

Johnston, Patricia Irwin. *Adopting after Infertility*. Indianapolis: Perspectives Press, 1992.

Kohn, Ingrid and Perry-Lynn Moffitt. *A Silent Sorrow: Pregnancy Loss*. New York: Delacorte, 1992.

Menning, Barbara Eck. *Infertility: A Guide for the Childless Couple*, Second Edition. New York: Prentice Hall, 1988.

RESOLVE, Inc. fact sheets. Somerville, MA.: RESOLVE, Inc.

Salzer, Linda. *Surviving Infertility: A Compassionate Guide through the Emotional Crisis of Infertility*. New York: HarperCollins, rev. 1991.

Shapiro, Constance Hoenk. *Infertility and Pregnancy Loss: A Guide for Helping Professionals*. San Francisco: Jossey-Bass, 1988.

Sifford, Darrell. *Only Child: Being One, Loving One, Understanding One, Raising One*. New York: Harper & Row, 1989.

Zoldbrod, Aline. *Men, Women and Infertility: Intervention and Treatment Strategies*. New York: Lexington Books, 1993.

Zoldbrod, Aline. *Getting Around the Boulder in the Road: Using Imagery to Cope with Fertility Problems*. Lexington, MA.: The Center for Reproductive Problems, 1990.

Notes

Chapter 1

1. A. F. Hanley, *Primary vs. Secondary Infertility*, RESOLVE fact sheet (Somerville, Mass.: RESOLVE, Inc., 1994), 1.

2. M. Beck and V. Quade, "Baby Blues: The Sequel," *Newsweek*, July 3, 1989, 62.

3. Carla Harkness, *The Infertility Book: A Comprehensive Medical and Emotional Guide* (Berkeley, Calif.: Celestial Arts, 1992), 77.

4. Beck and Quade, 62.

5. John Collins, Carol Rand, Elaine Wilson, William Wrixon, and Robert Casper, "The Better Prognosis in Secondary Infertility Is Associated with a Higher Proportion of Ovulation Disorders," *Fertility and Sterility* 45, no. 5 (May 1986):615.

Chapter 2

1. Group for the Advancement of Psychiatry, *The Joys and Sorrows of Parenthood* (New York: Charles Scribner & Sons, 1973), 82.

2. Anne Kelley Noone, "Hannah, Why Do You Weep? An Exploratory Study of the Adaptive Challenges Faced by Women Diagnosed with Premature Ovarian Failure" (unpublished master's thesis, Smith College, School of Social Work, 1994).

3. Barbara Eck Menning, *Infertility: A Guide for the Childless Couple*, 2nd ed. (Englewood Cliffs, N.J.: Prentice Hall, 1988), 114.

4. Noone, 55.

5. Susanne Morgan. *Coping with a Hysterectomy* (New York: Dial Press, 1982), 121.

6. Nadine Boehm, "No Brothers and Sisters for Zachary," *RESOLVE of Ohio Newsletter*, May 1989, Vol 9, No. 3 1–2.

7. Barbara Eck Menning, *Infertility: A Guide for the Childless Couple* (Englewood Clifts, N.J.: Prentice Hall, 1977) 117.

Chapter 3

1. Harriet Simons, "RESOLVE, Inc.: Advocacy within a Mutual Support Organization" (unpublished doctoral diss., Brandeis University, 1988), 181.

2.   Aline Zoldbrod, *Men, Women, and Infertility: Intervention and Treatment Strategies* (New York: Lexington Books, 1993), 19.

3.   Simons, 1988, 182.

4.   Zoldbrod, 19.

5.   Zoldbrod, 173.

6.   This discussion is adapated from the minutes of a RESOLVE of the Bay State meeting of support group leaders, compiled by Peg Beck.

7.   Jean Carter and Michael Carter, *Sweet Grapes: How to Stop Being Infertile and Start Living Again* (Indianapolis: Perspectives Press, 1989), 132–33.

Chapter 4

1.   Ingrid Kohn and Perry-Lynn Moffitt, *A Silent Sorrow: Pregnancy Loss* (New York: Delacorte, 1992), 222.

2.   Simons, 1988, 196.

3.   Kohn and Moffitt, 216.

4.   Miriam Mazor and Harriet Simons, Eds. *Infertility: Medical, Emotional, and Social Considerations* (New York: Human Sciences Press, 1984), 29.

5.   Zoldbrod, 61.

6.   Menning, 1988, 161.

7.   Kohn and Moffitt, 226.

8.   Menning, 1988, 162.

9.   Menning, 1988, 163.

10.   Patricia Mahlstedt and Page Johnson, *Coping with Infertility: How Family and Friends Can Help*, RESOLVE fact sheet (Somerville, Mass.: RESOLVE, Inc., revised 1994), 5.

Chapter 5

1.   Gjerde Dausch, "Secondary Infertility: A Personal Perspective," in *Primary vs. Secondary Infertility*, RESOLVE fact sheet (Somerville, Mass.: RESOLVE, Inc., May 1994), 2–3.

2.   Judith Calica, "Secondary Infertility: An Unexpected Disappointment," *Chicago Parent*, Oct. 1987, 8.

Chapter 6

1.   Anne Marie Murphy, "Parenting and Infertility," *Boston Parent's Paper*, January 1989, 5.

2.   John Defrain, Leona Martens, Jan Stork and Warren Stork, *Stillborn: The Invisible Death* (Lexington, Mass.: Lexington Books, 1986), 148.

3.   Patricia Irwin Johnston, *Taking Charge of Infertility* (Indianapolis: Perspectives Press, 1994), 237.

4.   Anne Bernstein, *Flight of the Stork: What Children Think (and When) about Sex and Family Building* Revised Edition (Indianapolis: Perspectives Press, 1994), 100, 166.

5. Murphy, 5.
6. Defrain et al., 149.
7. Earl Grollman, *Talking about Death* (Boston: Beacon Press, 1990), 2–3.
8. Johnston, 236, 237.
9. Defrain et al., 150.
10. Johnston, 244.
11. Defrain et al., 146.
12. Defrain et al., 143.
13. Grollman, 50, 78.
14. Defrain et al., 155.
15. Kohn and Moffitt, 238.
16. Harkness, 75.
17. Defrain et al., 153.
18. Defrain et al., 150.
19. Kohn and Moffitt, 238.
20. Fred Rogers and Clare O'Brien, *Mister Rogers Talks with Families about Divorce* (New York: Berkley Books, 1987).
21. Murphy, 5.
22. Rogers and O'Brien, 105.

Chapter 7

1. Boston Women's Health Book Collective, *Ourselves and Our Children* (New York: Random House, 1978), 30.
2. Boston Women's Health Book Collective, 31.
3. Martha Paci, "Pain as Real with One Child," in *Primary vs. Secondary Infertility*, RESOLVE fact sheet (Somerville, Mass.: 1994), 5.
4. Boston Women's Health Book Collective, 31.
5. Paci, 5–6.
6. Stephen Bank and Michael Kahn, *The Sibling Bond* (New York: Basic Books, 1982), 25.
7. Holly F. Simons, "Secondary Infertility," *Conceive Magazine*, May–June 1990, 15.
8. Lee Salk, *Familyhood* (New York: Simon & Schuster, 1992), 82.
9. Dausch, 3.
10. Dausch, 3.
11. Bank and Kahn, 26.
12. T. Berry Brazelton, *To Listen to a Child: Understanding the Normal Problems of Growing Up* (Reading, Mass: Addison-Wesley, 1984), 69–70.
13. Darrell Sifford, *Only Child: Being One, Loving One, Understanding One, Raising One* (New York: Harper & Row, 1989), 14.
14. Merle Bombardieri, *The Baby Decision: How to Make the Most Important Choice of Your Life.* (New York: Rawson Wade, 1981). 190–91.
15. Bank and Kahn, 27.
16. Brazelton, 76–77.
17. Sifford, 13.

18.   Louis Genevie and Eva Margolies, *The Motherhood Report: How Women Feel about Being Mothers* (New York: Macmillan, 1987), 66.
19.   Simons, 1990, 14.
20.   Defrain et al., 158–59.
21.   Harkness, 80.
22.   Simons, 1990 14.
23.   Harkness, 80.
24.   Dausch, 3.
25.   Kohn and Moffitt, 254–55.
26.   Kohn and Moffitt, 253.
27.   Sifford, 14.
28.   Harkness, 81.

Chapter 8

1.   Anne Marie Murphy, "Infertile Parents: A Silent Sorrow," *Boston Parent's Paper*, December 1988, 3.
2.   Murphy, 1988, 3.
3.   Murphy, 1988, 3.
4.   J. A. Collins, J. B. Garner, E. H. Wilson, W. Wrixon and R. Casper, "A Proportional Hazards Analysis of the Clinical Characteristics of Infertile Couples," *American Journal of Obstet. Gynecol.* Vol 148, Number 5 (March 1, 1984): 527–32.
5.   Kate Weinstein, *Living with Endometriosis* (Reading, Mass.: Addison-Wesley, 1987), 31.
6.   Weinstein, 32.
7.   Hanley, "Primary vs. Secondary Infertility," Resolve National Newsletter June 1990, 1.
8.   Weinstein, 31.
9.   Menning, 1988, xiv.
10.   Noone.

Chapter 9

1.   Genevie and Margolies, 284.
2.   Menning, 1977 146.
3.   Boehm, 1–2.
4.   Genevie and Margolies, 278–280.
5.   Carter and Carter, 14–15.
6.   Cooper, Susan and Ellen Glazer. *Beyond Infertility: The New Paths to Parenthood.* New York: Lexington Books, 1994, 108.

Chapter 10

1.   Carter and Carter, 48–49.
2.   Menning, 1988 170.
3.   RESOLVE National Newsletter. Summer 1994, Vol XIX, No. 3, 2.

4. Carter and Carter, 14–15.
5. Carter and Carter, 26–27.
6. Carter and Carter, 128.
7. Carter and Carter, 27.
8. Kohn and Moffitt, 295.
9. Simons, 1988, 180.

Index

Wanting Another Child

616.692   Simons, Harriet F.
SIM
          Wanting another
            child.

$23.00

DATE			